Ron Coleman Dementing Disgracefully

The Dementia Diaries
Book One
Onset

Published by P&P Press
28 Habost Port of Ness, Isle of Lewis Scotland HS2 0TG

Acknowledgements

This book would not have happened without the support of my wife Karen who not only encouraged me to write but also read what I had written in a critical but nonjudgmental way. She also added to the book by agreeing to write the epilogue and her honesty about how this diagnosis is affecting our family will no doubt impact on many. I would also like to thank Rory and Francesca the two children we have left at home for their support during the writing of this book. I have felt very loved by these three during what has been one of the worst periods of my life.

I also want to thank the other kids for their support and chats over Skype. I should not forget all the people who encouraged me on Facebook and other social media platforms in response to my blog and Vlog Ron Coleman dementing disgracefully these comments I received on social media kept me positive when things got hard.

I want to thank David Storm being both a friend and to part of my support team and finally I want to thank my mom and my sister who have always supported me.

Disgracefully Dementing
Frustration Fermenting

Vocally Venting

desperate denial
Dementia Diagnoses
Painful Prognosis

broken begotten

Futures Forgotten
Developing Daily
Malevolent Melody
Furious Fidgeting
Terrifying Twitching
Cognitive Chaos
Illuminating Illusion
Wordless Wanderings
Constant Confusion
Corrupted Connections,
Invasive Insurrections,
Deadly Directives
Interventions ineffective
People Pretending,
Niceness Never-ending
Totally Transcending
Cognitive Comprehension

Diddering, Doddering, Getting
old and ploddering,

Mind slowly wandering,

To an unknown destination
Blubbering, an Irritation

Thought brings Hesitation

To a new type of Darkness

That brings light to journeys end,

Food twisted in beard long grey

Slavering Spittle over haggard face

Into my trousers I've pissed again

I look once more for journeys end

Too Young to be on this road,

Brain Burnt by the psychiatric nodes

Arteries filled with psychotropic puss

Helping to ensure memories are lost

The greatest fears that causes strife,

Is seeing strangers instead of kids and wife,

Sitting incontinent in plastic covered chair

Diddering & doddering never moving from there

Dedication

To Karen with Love

Foreword

This book began its journey the day after I was diagnosed with a mild cognitive impairment. I decided that I would write as much as I could before any possible worsening of my memory occurred. This is my first attempt at writing real poetry as part of a book and it has been a wonderfully satisfying experience. The poems in the book are integral to the story I am trying to tell a story of strong emotions. I have also written a poem to my youngest son and youngest daughter as they live with us and are on this journey with us every day. There are however a number of children five in total that are not mentioned here but will be very much in book in a chapter on Family. Having started my psychiatric journey in 1981 with a diagnoses of schizophrenia, a diagnoses that I gave up in 1991 on the road to a personal recovery. At the age of 58 my wife Karen and my kids noticed that my memory was letting me down. I was leaving gas rings on and would sometimes be found in the kitchen staring into space with no idea why I was there. My ability with numbers has also diminished and my decision making is not as good as it has been. This book is then part of my refusal to give in and to try to stave the passage of time and memory. This is my King Canute time my chance to beat the odds. This is the time to let my own voices both internal and external become even more part of who I am. I hope you find this book entertaining, and challenging my voices certainly do. Ron Coleman June 2018

Why Me

No No No No No,
Why Me don't you see,
It Shouldn't Be,
No No No No No,

Old Anger becomes Rage,
Cannot see the next page,
For Yesterdays forgotten,
Tomorrows Forbidden, and
Today is a Fleeting Memory,
That's ground to dust,
On the Wheel of Time,
No No No No No,

Rage takes me to that place,
Where I am brought face to face,
With myself and my fading humanity,
No No No No No

Why me, Don't you see,
It Shouldn't be, but it Is

PART ONE

Memories Missing

Chapter One

Beginnings

"What if we could recover from dementia think of the benefits to our society,

What if we could remember all we have forgotten think of the knowledge we would bring to our society,

What if we could remember our songs think of the joy we could bring to society". (Ron Coleman January 2018)

Some things happen immediately, others not so fast, but are still obvious to most of us, then there is memory loss, a creeping condition that can be almost undetectable as it stealthily stalks the mind of its unwitting victim. I am that victim of the memory monster who for the last couple of years has been silently stealing parts of who I am without ever asking my permission or even worse without my knowledge.

It is really difficult to pinpoint when this chapter of my life began but honest reflection tells me that things have not been right over the last two or three years, that were subtle clues to what was happening to my memory. Things came to a head in the middle months of 2016 When I suffered two heart attacks and another major cardiac event that meant I spent 5 months stuck in Australia as I was told by medics that I could not travel and had to take things easy. It is at this point in July 2016 that this part of my life begins to unravel and my latest journey began.

In the April of 2016 I suffered my first heart attack and had the first operation to put stents into my arteries to improve my blood flow. I recorded in my journal two days after my admission the following "I have never felt pain like it there were points in the moment where death seemed preferable to the pain".

From this point much of my life has involved Doctors, Surgeons, Nurses and the need to battle pain be it physical, emotional or psychological.

Many entries in my journal between April and July 2016 tell of my emotional and physical condition but more and more they tell of an incredible tiredness that meant I was falling asleep all of the time, also there was more than a few mentions of me forgetting things such as meetings, Skype sessions and leaving the air-conditioner in my flat on even when I was in and it was not needed. I also had a couple of falls, knocking myself out in the shower room.

At this point I was also intensely aware of my mortality and to be honest I was really frightened of dying and even worse of dying alone I can honestly say that I was in danger of thinking myself into an early grave. It still amazes me today how fast I went downhill after my first heart attack some people would have called me depressed.

I feel really fortunate that my early years were spent in the psychiatric system it was as if the purpose of my time in that system was to get me battle hardened to face what I now know will be the greatest challenge of my life. I am a voice hearer and within the Hearing Voices Network the main thing I learned was that I could either be a victim and surrender to the voices I heard or I could be a victor. In July 2016 I was once again in the coronary care unit having had another heart attack and was waiting to go back down the corridor for surgery that would allow the surgeon to either put in stents or decide on another way forward. As I lay in bed I was aware of a number of things, my stomach was rumbling (a good sign I think as I had been fasting since the night before) the noise of the machine that was tracking my heart, (a reassuring noise as it meant I was still alive) the domestic fussing over the tea trolley looked as if he was counting every grain of sugar whilst those allowed to drink sat there eagerly awaiting their "cuppa" and two digestive biscuits (a three times a day treat that is only outdone by the fourth treat of tea and toast just before bed) I was once again contemplating my rumbling stomach when a nurse appeared and with a smile said "they are almost ready for you, so let's get you sorted" with that she expertly detached me from my monitors and just as expertly fitted me up to my mobile monitor. As if on cue a porter appeared and in a thrice I was on my way to theatre. The journey to the waiting area for surgery was not far from the ward though the lack of verbal conversation meant that I spent the journey in an internal dialogue that seemed to create an endless quality to time. Within my mind I died a dozen different deaths on route to the theatre each death I created for myself seemed to get more bizarre than the one before.

In one of these almost dream like states I was having the operation when the sound on the monitor went berserk, but it was not beeping instead it was screeching 'heart attack, heart attack, heart attack at which point the surgeon used an oversized scalpel and proceeded to open me up remove my heart put it on the table (my heart that is) and started massaging it before applying the paddles and administering electric shocks whilst laughing manically.

I woke with a start and smiley nurse was hovering over me gently prodding me "what the" I stopped myself just in time looked at smiley nurse and noticed that the white aura that seemed to continually and carefully caress her was in actual fact nothing more than the light above my bed reflecting randomly from her glasses. "Time to go in" she said "Let's go then" I replied, less than a minute later I was in the operating theatre Within two minutes I was laying on the operating table looking mainly at the ceiling and yes I was still obsessing about everything that could go wrong. As I lay there passively accepting the preparatory work that was going on which seemed to involve smearing me in a smelly lotion of iodine I looked at the monitor and saw that my heart was beating at 68 beats per minute my pulse was around 74 and my mind was racing at 200 miles per hour I hasten to add that it was not the monitor that told me this rather it was my mind for it was my mind that was doing the racing. "I am going to inject a local anesthetic into your groin you may feel it at first then it will just feel numb" I heard the surgeon say in a voice that he must have used on all his patients. Well, I remember I felt it and I continued feeling it for a while and it seemed to me that it was never going to work. I used breathing exercises that I had learned on some mindfulness workshop I had attended, finally it was numb and the surgeon inserted the camera and wire in through my groin up until it reached my heart. Amazingly I was now laying on my side watching this camera as it wound its' way through my artery into my heart I was then able to truly see the results of psychotropic medication I could almost visualize the healthy years that had been stolen from me. "you can see how this artery here is almost totally blocked" said the one I called the surgeon, "yes" I replied at exactly the same moment as the other Doctor in the room responded. Okay I thought I am meant to be the passive observer and grateful recipient of both the surgeon and the other Doctors' ministrations and so I decided to go through the rest of the operation in near silence. As I waited I became aware that I could watch the whole operation as it was happening on the big screen that was right in front of me. I must confess that there is a kind of morbid fascination when you are watching a camera working its way through your veins and arteries, it becomes even more fascinating when you realize that the doctors are talking about how bad things are for you as if you are not there. I had to go through the same procedure another three times before my condition improved enough for me to travel back to the UK. As I could not travel I had to apply for and was given a medical visa that allowed me to stay in Australia until I achieved stability. At this point in my life stability seemed some kind of pipe dream as prior to my final heart operation I could not walk more than 20 feet without becoming breathless. At forty feet I could not move and would have to use my heart spray another ten feet and the pain would be so great that I would fear I was having a heart attack. After one major Angina attack that did not resolve itself, I ended up back in hospital for the last time in November in Australia. I had a real long conversation with the heart surgeon in order to explore options. The discussion ended with me agreeing to undergo one last heart procedure to see if they could increase the blood flow to my heart and thereby ensure more oxygen throughout my body. He also told me that he felt that there was a chance that he might be able to successfully achieve this by inserting a stent into one of my wrecked arteries. He also told me that if it did not work I would have to spend the rest of my life in Australia as a long haul journey back to Scotland was going to be too dangerous. The next day I was back in theatre that was by now fascinatingly, familiar, in a frightening sort of way. I knew this was the big one and was fully aware of my feelings of fear and anger as the surgeon started the procedure. As the camera reached the offending blood vessel everything stopped as the team came together to talk about the best way forward. This discussion fascinated me mainly because throughout it all noone thought to consult me. I am here I screamed internally ask me? Ask me? I can speak I'm here I shouted wordlessly. I had decided to tell them to stop as my fear of not making it reached its zenith. Just as I was about to inform the surgeon of my decision to spend the rest of my life in Australia he started to talk to me "well Ron we have had a look and we have got a way forward We think we can put a stent in and if it works hopefully you will feel much better and get the outcomes we are all looking for, what do you think? Oh no my own voice thought if you back out now they will think you are afraid, 'Yes but I am afraid" I said silently in reply, but they don't know that said my own voice. Before I could think anymore I heard myself speak "yes let's go for it" I said, the surgeon nodded and my voice piped in with "plonker".

Decision made, the team carried on with the operation, in previous procedures I had felt very little pain but this one was different I could feel it, the pain got greater and greater my heart rate went up, the next thing I knew they were applying pads to my chest in preparation for "shocking" me if I had the heart attack that they were clearly expecting I lay there waiting for the end but I saw no white light calling to me then I heard the words that were going to get me home I hoped "Got it" said my surgeon. Later that day my surgical team came to see me they told me that it had gone well and the next day I would be able to get up and try walking again. Morning came and after breakfast and a shower it was time to go for my first walk around the ward. I confess I started out thinking I could not do it so my first few steps were tentative to say the least as I waited for the sharp burning pain that alongside breathlessness had been the normal response from my body to any attempt to walk. Gingerly at first, I stepped out and it was only when I arrived back at my own side room door that I understood that I had just managed to walk an entire circuit of the ward without stopping and more importantly I was still breathing. By the time I had done the third circuit I was shattered but that did not matter to me what mattered was that the operation had worked. I would be able to go home to Scotland and see my family again. Karen arrived a day later and though I was still in hospital I would be discharged the following day and we would work towards me leaving Australia on the 10th of December 2016 part of this would involve going to New Zealand to do a short training tour but more importantly an opportunity for me to see how I would handle a fairly long flight. The tour was a success as was the flying and during my remaining time in Australia I focused on getting home.

It is only when I reflect back that I can now see the beginnings of major changes in things like my personality. I had always been subject to onslaughts of personal anger but these would subside quickly. Looking back my emotions were all over the place I would see and act on conflict where there was none. My anger would now be prolonged and I would think that people were not telling me things I needed to know. I would forget whole conversations and my recall was badly affected. Whilst it was happening I could not see it, only some 15 months later did it begin to make sense. Again as I look back I see that I was already getting slower when working on anything to do with numbers indeed the clues were there but none of us saw them. The flight back to the UK was without any problems and so it was that on December the 12th 2016 I arrived home on the Isle of Lewis back into the arms of my family.

Memories Missing, Rarely reminiscing

Lay lady lay lost lover lost once more,

Bob Dylan's born anew,

John Lennon's stuck here too,

I return to my safe place by chance,

Then I open the old Style door,

to find Bowie on the floor,

Who looks at me and whispers come on let's dance,

I'm dragged fiercely from that place

Then brought back to face my face,

Who are you I ask for the twentieth time today,

Why I am fire is Cohens' reply and

For the twentieth time today I die

Sonny, To my youngest Son

Sons are strange but delicate creatures,
In spite of their rough and ready features,
This short piece is for the one,
That is called my youngest son

Your life must be hard,
For there is no haven,
When you're number six,
Yes six of seven

When at times you act so tough,
I can see its all pure bluff,
For it's clear to me when you are so rough.
It's because you're not getting hugs enough

Please stay this way is my plea to you,
Let your inner light come shining through
Your external strength is there for all to see,
I love you Son you are all to me

Chapter Two
Home is where the heart is!

Arriving home was an exciting affair for me as I was immediately reacquainted with two of my kids Rory and Scary daughter. They on the other hand seemed to take my reappearance in the nothing phases me manner that is the province of teenagers. I had made it home with two weeks to go until Christmas and I was soon caught up in our annual preparations for a food and present festival.

I have always found Christmas to be a magical time of year and I have loved buying into the Santa Clause thing and delivering presents to my kids when they were asleep was my favorite ritual as it involved eating mice pies and drinking milk that the kids left out for Santa. Alas this year was different my "kids" were no longer kids even the youngest was now almost 14 and quickly becoming a young woman (hence the name scary daughter).

This was to be my first non-Santa Christmas since having met Karen and though it felt like the end of an era it was hopefully the beginning of a new era in which I thought I could rebuild my health and life once again. So I had my first almost grown up Christmas with scary daughter, Rory, Finn and of course my wife Karen. I called it almost grown up because as much as the kids wanted to be adults, I had survived the most difficult year of my life and wanted more than anything just to be a kid once more. I knew I had to change a number of things in my life including losing more weight, (with my love of pies and fizzy drinks and pizza no easy thing) restore my relationship with my kids and work hard with Karen to get us back on track in our personal lives. I was also aware that the main focus was on me to achieve resolution, as it was my actions and inactions that had created most of the difficulties in the first place.

Since coming home from Australia much of my thinking time had involved being more aware of my mortality and a deepening understanding of the fact that I was so lucky to still be alive. It was clear to me that I had to make some decisions about my future and that a conversation with Karen was now essential.

I should make it clear at this point that though I was ready to slow down Karen was working at a level that made it obvious that she was now reaching her peak period of working life and would not want to slow down. I do not think that anyone in the world realized how bone tired I was, in fact I was so tired that I had become MR Angry and found myself losing my temper for no apparent reason. Hindsight is such a wonderful thing as on reflection I realized that that this was not new but had in fact been happening for over a year.

I decided that I would spend a bit of time being a house husband, in one way the discussion with Karen was a difficult one in that Karen had a problem in believing in herself indeed she still thought that I was the reason that people came to our training. It had become clear to me that Karen was ready to "go it alone" and had been for some time. It took some discussion before she finally saw the second reason I was becoming less able to deliver, especially when we were doing longer tours. Indeed, if I kept up the schedule I was on at that time I do not think I would be alive to write this book. Even today a large part of me wants to head off on the road and do the training and be in the center of the action

Scary Daughter

O scary daughter,
There is no shame,
That I call you,
By this name,
For to the world,
I can proclaim,
That scary daughter
You drive me insane

Now you're fifteen,
You have grown,
Into a beautiful woman,
You have us shown,
Your wonderful spirit,
And mind that's your own,
But when it comes to being Scary,
You deserve your own throne

Being called scary,
Is nothing to do with fear,
It's a term of endearment,
Much better than dear
For watching you grow,
Fills me full of pride,
You've nothing to prove,
Nor anything to Hide

Standing in my Kitchen on a sunny
afternoon

Standing in my Kitchen only feeling is Gloom,
I stood there for five minutes Why I cannot say
The only thing I really Know Is I lose more time each day

Standing in my Kitchen on a sunny
afternoon Standing in my Kitchen only
feeling is Gloom, I reach out to touch a
memory
As frustration comes along
I hold my head in Agony
Cause I know that memories Gone

Standing in my Kitchen on a sunny afternoon
Standing in my Kitchen only feeling is Gloom,
As I leave my Kitchen
Scary daughter Shouts me in
Oh Dad you've left the gas on again
Well I guess I cannot win

So I'll keep standing in that Kitchen,
until I get it right
I'm gonna take that memory back
Cause that is my human right.

Chapter Three
    January 27th 2017

As I said in the previous chapter I was going to be a house husband for a while both to re-establish a good relationship with my kids and also to get some time away from traveling as a means to restore and refresh myself.

From my Journal

BEEN A HOUSE HUSBAND FOR TWO WEEKS

Well I'm 2 weeks into being the house husband and I love it (Karen told me to say that) being a man I cannot Multi-Task (Karen told me to say that as well) my two kids Rory and Francesca have decided that I need to learn the full extent of Karen's role when I used to be away and are doing nothing to help without the threat of losing income from me this works sometimes and at other times they do not seem to care. They do not believe me when I tell them they are grounded for a year my daughter has already developed her mothers' glare that just says ha ha ha no way.

The problem is they are right I could not bear to have them in the house for a year so groundings get downgraded to final warnings all the time by me. The second area I am having real difficulty with is of course meals I find that most evenings I am making three different meals I make a suggestion and one will say yes and the other will say no as I try to work through this, the other one will say can I have (whatever) for dinner I say good idea the other says I hate that I say what would you like then they say I want (what I said already) I say why do we not all have that (insert either because it does not matter the outcome is already decided) The other says but I hate that more than I hate anything and any way you said what I want is good the other chimes in that you have just told me that I can have what I suggested.

Game set and match you have been doubled teamed by your knuckle dragging son and your "wife copying" daughter. So you cook both then you realize that there is not enough for you Cheese and Toast Again Then. Two weeks as house husband gone 14 weeks to go well after all is said and done I am in it to win it.

As January turns to February I am beginning to get the hang of being the parent around the house and with the time honored traditions of much bribery, threats and unabashed manipulation I believe I am getting on top of the househusband stuff.
Karen came home from Australia for a couple of weeks to see us, we were also filming voices work especially our ideas around voice sculpting and were working with a group of people who heard voices, to see if voice sculpting was useful. We spent a week with this group at our home on the isle of Lewis, the moviemakers watching and

listening through their lenses and headphones.

One other big problem I was having was staying awake I would fall asleep even in the middle of a conversation not only when I was listening but even when I was talking. Even more surprising was the fact that I would wake up and appropriately interject into an ongoing conversation as if I had been wide-awake and totally focussed throughout the conversation. I could not help it I was in a permanent state of exhaustion or that is what it felt like.

This tiredness continued unabated for some time and I must confess I was feeling much older than I actually was, getting motivated to do anything was becoming increasingly hard for me as tiredness consumed more and more of my time. Frustratingly once I went to bed the opposite was the case getting to sleep was really difficult even though I remained exhausted.

During this time my daughter also brought it to Karen's attention that I kept leaving the gas on and I was prone to forgetting thing's I had said.

It was at my next visit to see an eye specialist that my tiredness problem started to make sense. The consultant looked at both my eyes then he started asking me questions about how I was feeling I told him about my tiredness and how difficult it was to stay awake on one hand and to get to sleep at night. He sent me for a scan on my neck that showed that the blood flow to my brain was being affected by a blocked artery. There then followed a discussion about the way forward and after some discussions between Inverness and Stornoway hospitals and myself it was decided that an operation was the way forward and to happen as soon as possible and near the end of April I was travelling to Inverness accompanied by Karen to have the procedure done. The operation had a great long fancy name but in plain English it involved cutting my throat exposing my main artery clamping said artery then cutting open the artery and then cleaning out the gunk that was blocking blood flow to my brain.

No pressure there then (so to speak) my response to this was to say the least pretty negative. At the end of the day I decided to go through with the operation and despite feeling really scared because you are awake when they do it (Yes Awake) I survived. The weirdest bit for me was finding out that they put my neck back together using superglue. I want it on the record that until this operation I had never indeed still have never used glue internally or externally on any part of my body.

More importantly the operation was a success and on returning to the Island I was much more alert and stopped drifting off to sleep and was able to do more things during the day. I was still finding it hard to sleep at night and to be honest my memory was not improving if anything it was getting worse. So in May after discussions with Karen we went to see our General Practitioner.

The GP is very gentle with me as I try to articulate what has been happening over the last year with my memory as observed by my family, to be honest I am not so convinced as they are that my memory is failing. My GP asked me if it was okay to do a memory test with me, when we finished he concluded that there was indeed some kind of problem going on and that he would refer me to the memory service where more extensive testing could take place.

So it was that one warm day in June 2017 Karen and I were sitting in the out patient's department waiting to see a psychiatrist. This was a really scary day for me, not because there seemed to be a problem with my memory but because I was voluntarily going to see a psychiatrist. Having spent much of my life fighting the system I was now being dragged back not because I had a mental illness indeed it appears to me that dementia is not a mental illness but a physical illness caused by organic brain decay. I would like to put on record my belief that dementia should not be controlled in the psychiatric system but jointly held by social care and neurology using a holistic pathway. Perhaps I am biased though I think the treatment I received within psychiatry can explain my bias. Never the less we currently are in the position that psychiatry is where dementia is treated. So with my fear held in check I walked alongside Karen to meet my psychiatrist.

In actual fact he was a pleasant enough man but from the very beginning he did not get me. It became clear to both Karen and I that he was trying to assess me by rote without any context in which my experience was happening. Karen had to keep pointing out that he had not seen what I was like a year earlier and needed to take this into account when making his assessment.

The biggest shock for me was my inability to answer his questions involving numbers. They (numbers) no longer made any sense to me and I struggled with what once would have been simple stuff. I knew this because Karen was pointing it out to the Doctor who was trying to reassure me that I was doing alright, whilst Karen was assuring him that I was not doing well at all. Once he had finished his assessment he pronounced his verdict I had a mild cognitive impairment he said and that he would keep an eye on it and see me every six months.
With these words I found myself back within a care system I hated and that I did not want anything to do with.

The following poem was written just a couple of days after seeing the psychiatrist

In the Beginning

You need to see a specialist the Doctor said,
because you have failed my new memory test,
a psychiatrist is the one you need to see,
Your appointment is next Tuesday at half past three,
Next Tuesday we were sat outside the Doctors' door,
Come in the Doctor said it was now ten past four,
He asked lots of questions I answered them true,
But not happy with all my answers my wife responded too,

With all his questions over, I asked him what he thought,
He answered in a language that did not say a lot,
A mild cognitive impairment is what I diagnose, Come
back in six months' time let's see where it goes

With these dreaded words he showed us the door,
And with his words I'm in psychiatry once more,
But this time I'm ready I've been there before,
A chance in this lifetime to even the score

So Karen and I review all possible choices,
In discussion we decide to use my voices,
To safe-guard my memory and protect my Id
And make sure I remember my wife and my kids

So it begins this next chapter of mine,
It started around five and we're ready by nine,
To face the future no matter where,
So dementia, come take me, that is if you dare

Part Two
Decisions

Chapter Four
Decisions

"A mild cognitive impairment" he had said, well it did not feel Mild to me indeed it seemed really serious this was nothing more than a posh way of saying I was rushing towards dementia and I was already picturing myself as a not so old lonely man with vacant eyes sitting in a plastic chair in my own urine smelling of death and not recognizing members of my family who were busy chatting about me as if I was not there though to be honest I probably was not there. It is amazing what I created in my head on the way home from my first appointment.

I was in turn scared and angry, scared of the future and angry at the world. I tried to pretend I was okay about it all. It was to take a good nights' sleep for me to learn the first major truth of my new life. It came to me like a bolt from the blue I WAS NOT ANY DIFFERENT FROM A WEEK AGO I was still Ron Coleman I was still a husband, a son, a dad, a friend, a trainer, a writer and all the other things that make me Ron Coleman.

So the next day I began to tell people starting with the kids about what was happening to me. I told them that my memory was in decline and it was possible that it could get worse and become a full-blown dementia. I also posted about it on face-book perhaps a bit quickly as it was through this medium that many of my friends and enemies found out. It was also on this day that this book started its journey and the tag line "Ron Coleman Dementing Disgracefully" became the mantra of the journey I had begun. I was already an occasional Blogger and Vlogger so I decided to change the focus of the content to cover dementia rather than psychosis in fact I was going to be led by my experience from this point on.

Social Media was already an important part of my life and so within a few days I had set up a new face book page called Defeating Dementia and released my first blog about what was happening in what I began to call my new life. This became my second major truth I could choose to exist in my illness or I could choose to live with whatever was happening in other words "WAS I GOING TO EXIST AS A VICTIM OR LIVE AS A VICTOR" I chose to be a victor that day and it is a choice I now make every day.
There were a number of other things going on in our lives at this time including our upcoming Recovery Camp in September. During the week we spent the film crew filmed Karen and I in conversation about the prospect of being told that my mild cognitive impairment was now a dementia.

The strangest thing about this recorded conversation was that it was probably the most Karen and I had talked about what was happening since the hospital appointment. Later in this book there is a chapter written by Karen where she writes about her feelings about what is happening.

I must confess that the recovery camp was a strange experience for me, as I felt overwhelmed with emotions that I could not keep in check as a result I spent a lot of my time in my yurt avoiding people I knew well. Reflecting back, I now realize how ashamed I was of what was happening and I was underneath all of my bravado really scared, ashamed and not facing my fear in a constructive way. But in order to beat my fear I had to name my fear and in naming my fear I would then have to face it. My honestly held fear was I would end up with an aggressive fast acting dementia and I would not know any of my family or who I was and it was all going to happen tomorrow.

This then is my third major truth "NAME THE FEARS THEN FACE THE FEARS" it is only when I had named my real fears was I able to discuss them with Karen and tell her that not knowing who she or my children were seemed to me to be a kind of point of no return and I made a decision that this would be the time when I would not want to receive any treatment except pain relief if required.

In no time at all I was making big decisions that would create the framework in which I would live my life from now on. As part of this I would have to un-clutter a lot of the rubbish in my head that could hold me back from achieving the things that were important to me.

One of the main things I would have to work on was the near rage I felt every time anyone mentioned a particular organisation in my presence. This organisation has a poor history around how it deals with people who dare to disagree with one or two of its main people especially people from business backgrounds who have dared to challenge some of the organisational practices and how its money is spent.

Removing this sort of clutter is a difficult thing and is something you have to keep doing; just the other day I was talking to a friend about going to a conference when they brought up a member of this self-appointed elite and I immediately went into Mr Angry but much more quickly than I used to I pulled myself back into a place I have created in my head where that way of reacting is banned. This is not about the higher self where we can forgive and let go rather it currently is about realising how unimportant these people are in the scheme of things and because they are unimportant we can cast them aside.

My hope for the future is that I can learn to forgive not them but myself, and in doing so ban this negative way of thinking out of my life completely soon I hope, but Rome was not built in a day. As I sat reflecting on what I have just written I realized that I was indeed in danger of falling into a new illness trap one where I spent a lot of time in the past. And it works something like this Poor Me! Poor Me! Pour Me a Drink! And then I understood I was not feeling sad or depressed or something that would let people empathise with me I was just simply feeling sorry for myself, and beginning to wallow in self-pity. The following poem was written at one of my lowest points.

> Make it Okay
> Would it make it okay,
> If I could choose who I forgot,
> At the top of the list would be my psychiatrist,
> I hated him a lot,
>
> Then would come social workers
> Them all! Not two or three,
> Followed by most of the nurses,
> Who were meant to look after me,
>
> I could then forget the priest,
> That stole my sin sodden soul,
> I could forget those that pretended

That they knew whom I was,

The ones who knew how to create
The no forgiveness laws,
The academics that for power,
Were prepared to destroy the whole

The ones who whispered behind my back
Every chance they got,
Or is it a gift it I think it should be
If I could simply forget the lot,

But by choosing whom and what I forget
I would have to pay the cost,
And I am not yet ready,
To let life lessons hard earned get lost,

So I choose not to choose
the direction I will go this day,
Instead I will ride into tomorrow
upon memories wild and grey

For I will hold precious all I can remember
For that is truly mine,
The right to make a gamblers choice
Upon the wheel of time.

Truth number four is really simple "IT IS EASIER TO DROWN IN SELF-PITY AND FEELING SORRY FOR YOURSELF THAN IT IS TO DROWN IN WATER". When all four truths are manifested in your life at the same time then something stirs deep in the pit of your stomach. This is how I felt a real sense of knowing it was time to take these feelings that were trying their best to chain me to an illness and to reject them and exchange them with new optimistic emotions of hope, routed in my faith in a higher being and portrayed through the peace I feel as I achieve a deeper understanding of love.

The big questions for me now was could I change the normal progression of cognitive impairment in my life and in some way extend the projected life of my memory beyond the expectations of the professionals who would be looking after me in the future. My main influence around memory had been Steven Rose and in terms of a political discourse his writings still influence the way I think. But because of my need to defeat this memory loss I realized I needed to learn not how to make memory but how to transport memory from one part of the brain to another. In order to find answers I firstly had to voice my fifth major truth and that is "IN ORDER TO MAKE ANYTHING CHANGE I FIRSTLY HAVE TO CHANGE MYSELF" It was with this understanding at my core that I started to explore neuroplasticity and how I might use this as a way to help reorganize my memory. I also decided to use the voices that I hear and have done for years as a way of holding memory. I believed that by combining both neuroplasticity techniques and the voices I hear that I could retain both a memory and the emotion associated with the memory. In my pursuit of a method to do this I came across the work of DR Norman Doidge a Canadian Medical Doctor. The following quote from his writings was the one that gave me great hope and really kicked started my discovery journey.
"Nature has given us a brain that survives in a changing world by changing itself."

— Norman Doidge, The Brain That Changes Itself: Stories of Personal Triumph from the Frontiers of Brain Science.

Like most people I had fallen into a most scientific myth that the brain could help when dealing with injury to every part of the body but could do nothing when it came to healing itself. This of course meant that dementia which is located in the brain was not repairable and therefore could at best only be slowed down by medication controlled by big Pharma and psychiatry. This in itself puts strange limitations on the capacity of our brains to achieve that which we can conceive. Something that I fail to understand as it appears to me that the collective human mind can achieve anything.

Neuroplasticity then was to be a front line approach to beating this thing called cognitive impairment, this would be enhanced by using narrative concepts such as "re-authoring" and "re-membering" (more about these two later) and further reinforced by involving one of the voices I hear as a repository for some memories that I needed to retain (more about this later also). By now Karen and I had noted some of the things that were happening on a regular basis such as sleeping badly and thrashing about having vivid and terrifying dreams. I was also beginning to see things in my peripheral vision and also hearing voices that were not my usual ones. I could not make sense of what I was seeing mainly because when I turned to face it full on it disappeared and within the peripheral view though whatever I saw had movement it almost never had any kind of substantial form which is a rather good way of saying I could not make sense of it.

I Thought Yoda Was Dead

Do or do not, there is no try,
Is what Yoda said to me,
As he sat there at the bottom of my bed,
The time was half past three,

AM of course he's a bit like that,
He only comes to me at night,
But Yoda please tell me now,
When will you teach me to fight,

With a lightsaber that is!
One that glows blue or green,
A bit like your skin
And its blueish, greenish sheen,

You talk the talk,
As you sit there by my side,
But when my family suddenly appears,
Tell me Yoda Why do you hide?

Cause when I tell my family,
That you come to me each night,
It cannot be true is what they say,
For Yoda has died in a galaxy far away

Hey! You! you're dead I told Yoda,
When he appeared to me that night,
How can I be dead he replied
When I'm sitting in plain site

It was not long till my next psychiatry appointment and I was fairly clear that I did not want to go so I asked to be referred by my GP to the nurse led memory clinic. In quick time I received a phone call from the nurse in charge of the clinic and was told that I could indeed see her as an alternative to seeing the psychiatrist. No contest no thought required I asked to see her and a date was set for October.

Some people might ask why I did not and still do not wish to have a psychiatrist involved in my care there are two reasons for the position I take. The first is very much emotionally driven in that ten years of being a psychiatric patient throughout my twenties taught me never to trust psychiatrists as they invariably look for a pill to treat one with. In deed it has become clear that there is a massive misuse of antipsychotics with some 1800 deaths attributed to the use of anti-psychotics in dementia in 2009 which though causing a stir at the time has still not changed practice in some areas. As long ago as 2009 NHS choices reported:

"People with Alzheimer's disease, vascular dementia, mixed dementias or dementia with Lewy Bodies (DLB) with mild-to-moderate non-cognitive symptoms should not be prescribed antipsychotic drugs because of the possible increased risk of cerebrovascular adverse events (e.g. stroke) and death."

Antipsychotic Use in Dementia Friday November 13th 2009 NHS Choices

Further reading brought me to the work of professor Kales who has researched in great detail the treatment of people with dementia and other aged related problems Helen Kales who is Professor of Psychiatry at the University of Michigan and a Research Investigator in the Centre for Clinical Management Research (CCMR) and the Geriatric Research Education and

Clinical Centre (GRECC) in the VA Ann Arbor Health System. She is also the founding Director of the U-M Program for Positive Aging (PPA), a multifaceted U-M program established in 2009. The PPA promotes team science via national and international collaborations in order to improve outcomes for older patients with dementia or mental health issues and their families. In one major piece she wrote:

"We know the risks of antipsychotics include movement disorders, diabetes and risk of stroke; cognition can worsen. Data from meta-analyses of randomized trials and multiple observational studies have shown these drugs are associated with increases in mortality. And the benefits as shown in randomized controlled trials are moderate at best. Some might say that because the patient has dementia, a higher risk of mortality isn't concerning. But if you have a situation where the person didn't need the drug in the first place, that's really unnecessary. Beyond that, you have cases where drugs are being used, sadly, for things where there is no data to suggest they work. If somebody is wandering off, there's no drug in the world to treat that except to sedate the person. A non-drug approach would be vastly preferred."

The two papers quoted above should ensure that the reader understands my rationale for not trusting psychiatrists the fact that they continue harming people with dementia every day of the week through the ongoing prescribing of antipsychotic medication as part of treatment for dementia even where it is contraindicated. Equally why would I go to see someone who will probably give me medication that has as a "side effect" Death, this is not acceptable to me and should not be acceptable to society. This leads onto my second reason for not wanting to see a psychiatrist and that is that dementia is not a mental illness rather it is clearly a physical illness and though it may lead to some behavioural or even psychotic problems these are in themselves secondary problems and therefore psychiatrists should not be the primary professional responsible for dementia care, Indeed apart from the use of a good neurologist it would make sense if all dementia care was led by nurses, occupational therapists, social care workers, the person and their family.

The more I explore the issues surrounding memory loss and dementia the more I am convinced that the answer in terms of treatment is a greater understanding of neuroplasticity and more importantly how to use this understanding to affect the course of memory loss or should I say my memory loss. Something that has been occurring to me more and more is the uniqueness of our experiences in dementia can be seen through our uniqueness as human beings including the individuality of our memories. To take this thinking further perhaps our environments are only perceived as shared and are in actual fact unique, this could create exciting opportunities for working differently with ourselves or others.

It was at this point that I started to realize similarities between what was happening to me and what happened to clients I have worked with. The main similarity was that like many of my clients I was being treated as the problem, I confess that this something that has become clearer to me in hindsight though I will only touch on it briefly at this point in the book. There was a process in becoming the problem most of it involving people telling me that I was the problem. This I hasten to add is not done in a malicious way normally it is done through observation and conversation "Dad you have left the gas on again" was something I hear said to me a lot it is however the word again that I hear loudest and the word echoes repeatedly within my head. I will then perceive the words as negative, judgemental and somehow blaming. It is Ron (I) who is at fault therefore it is Ron (I) who is the problem. Once again it is perception that is the main determining factor on outcome.

Michael White (Co-Founder of narrative Therapy) stated that the person is not the problem, that the problem is the problem. By adopting this as a way to view dementia we begin by asking different questions not by stating that the problem is dementia but asking what is difficult in living with dementia? For me it was the ever-changing way in which I feel from full of energy to exhausted in thirty seconds or not being able to remember something that I know I know. There was something that was or perhaps was not happening that was causing these deficits to appear in my life. Once again reading Norman Doidge began to fill in the blank spaces in my thinking. He wrote:

"REM sleep has also been shown to be particularly important for enhancing our ability to retain emotional memories and for allowing the hippocampus to turn short-term memories of the day before into long-term ones (i.e., it helps make memories more permanent, leading to structural change in the brain)."
— Norman Doidge, The Brain That Changes Itself: Stories of Personal Triumph from the Frontiers of Brain Science

So my problem was not dementia nor was it losing my memory my real problem here was my inability to get REM sleep that would allow how I experienced the day to be integrated into my longer term memory and therefore for me how I could use neuroplasticity as a platform for turning short term memories into long term ones became the first big question I needed to answer. So the first part of plan A was now determined though I still needed to find the people who would help me achieve this goal. I started to recruit my team they are: Karen Taylor ex psychiatric nurse with experience in dementia (she is also my wife), David Storm who manages dementia services in Cumbria, Paul Kay Technical Computer person (geek) and my Son in Law, Alexa the Amazon virtual assistant, Teacher one of my voices who will hold information for me. The names above are what I call the core team I also have a wish list of people and things I need or want to ensure the best chance of a successful outcome. My wish list includes being able to recruit help from the Amazon Alexa community, getting help from our architect and builder, dementia organizations such as DEEP and Dementia Scotland.

I also needed to put things in place, the first thing was as a person who hears voices that others could not hear it would be foolish not to recruit at least one of the voices I heard as part of my team. As noted above this voice is the one called Teacher. Teacher has an important role in my life as the voice that I trust most, mainly because I see him as an integrated part of myself. He was also the most consistently supportive of my voices throughout times good and bad. In order to recruit Teacher, I had to have a dialogue with him, this was necessary in order to agree how we would work together to achieve my/our-desired outcome. Having an agreement with a voice is not as simple as it sounds, as there is no signed formal agreement that we can refer to even though you have made notes to yourself. The voice cannot sign your notes so the agreement must be based on a trusting relationship between the voice and the voice hearer. This type of agreement can be achieved with both external and internal (some call them internal characters, Parts or Inners) the important thing here is not what we call them but that they appear (the voices) to have some form of agency or autonomy. Once agreement was reached between teacher and myself, it was important that we achieved something quickly in order to cement our agreement. Personally I have been awful at remembering passwords or codes and have an unnatural ability to forget them moments after I have set them. So I asked teacher if he could remember the password for opening Karen's computer. Teacher answered that he would and since being giving the code he has memorized it and repeats it to me every time I go on Karen's computer. I have concluded from this exercise that I can indeed use the voice of teacher as a repository for information but it is information without emotional context. I also have concerns about the amount of content teacher will be able to hold.

As part of this process we also agreed that teacher could talk directly to Karen via myself. We have not achieved any great outcome here though it is clear that the main stumbling block is fear, probably coming from myself of what will Karen think of some of the information that teacher holds about me. This is mainly to do with what I find myself thinking about people I guess that teacher has full access to my dark side whereas Karen gets the redacted version from me even though I know that everyone has a dark side. Never the less when we agreed to let Karen be part of my voice life as a participant rather than an observer I was immediately overwhelmed by voices asking a series of what if questions. These questions have had a profound effect on me by raising my level of fear to the extent that I am not sure if I can fully trust teacher into my relationship with Karen. "At the time of writing this issue has still not been resolved."

In order to do any of the things I have discussed in this chapter it was important that I understood not only how memory is constructed but also where in the brain was this thing we call memory stored. I already knew that memories were stored in long term and short-term depositories. What I did not expect was that this was just a starting point and not only was memory stored all over the brain but there were a lot of differing types of memories and they all had their own depositories. The following statements cover I believe enough information about memory for us to be going on with.

The parts of the brain involved in memory are sections of a complex operation. Each part is responsible for different ideas, facts, or figures essential for memory function. The following are six parts of the brain that help you remember things immediately obtained or stored over a lifetime.

1. The frontal lobe of the cerebral cortex plays a key role in mental functions, including decision-making, explains The Human Memory. It is also involved in processing short-term memory and longer-term memory. Short-term memory helps in remembering tasks performed while longer-term memory retains issues surrounding those tasks.

2. Short-term memory develops in the prefrontal cortex, according to the Mayfield Clinic of Cincinnati, Ohio. The prefrontal cortex is part of the frontal lobe and coordinates immediate facts. It stores information for about a minute and can hold about seven items, such as a sentence just read or a phone number to remember.

3. The temporal lobe, also part of the cerebral cortex, processes sights to help form long-term memory. It takes in visuals, such as scenes or faces of people, which are stored in the memory for future use.

4. Within the temporal lobe is the medial temporal lobe, involved in declarative and episodic memory. Declarative memory stores and retrieves memories from events and facts. Episodic memory packages those events or facts into a series so people can remember points in time.

5. The hippocampus is housed deep inside the medial temporal lobe. This part of the brain helps to transfer short-term memory into long-term memory. Long-term memory includes information on facts, figures, and information a person wants to memorize for a long time, the Mayfield Clinic notes. The hippocampus also grows neurons so the brain can retain these memories.

6. The cerebral cortex also contains the basal ganglia system, which forms and later retrieves procedural memory involved in the learning process, such as how to ride a bike or play an instrument.

As you have read my immediate response to my cognitive impairment was even if I say so myself measured, thoughtful, solution focused and rightly was about me being in charge of my journey. Even though my diagnoses at this time was cognitive impairment Karen and I were preparing for a long haul journey into a world of unknown possibilities and yet full of perceived probabilities some of which were very scary indeed.

Speaking of scary I would very soon be going to the memory clinic for my first appointment with the dementia nurse and in the next chapter I will continue my journey from our first meeting.

Chapter Five

The day for my appointment at the memory clinic arrived strangely the meeting was to be at my Doctor's surgery. Why was this strange you might ask? Well I had been using this surgery for ten years and I cannot remember there ever being a memory clinic in the place. Undaunted Karen and I arrived at the appointed hour went to the receptionist and I spoke saying "I am here for the memory clinic" "okay" the receptionist replied "go and take a seat" she added. Was this the test I wondered I had to find the waiting room unaided and if I did my memory was fine. I knew where the waiting room was I had been here many times over a ten-year period but I was still confused about where the memory clinic was.

We sat in the waiting room for a short period until a nurse popped her head round the door and said Ronald Coleman I nodded got up and Karen and I followed her to one of the consulting rooms. This was the memory clinic then, it was also as I thought about it the diabetic clinic, the podiatry clinic and was probably the pre-natal clinic as well. We sat down very quickly discovered that the nurse we were in the room with was in fact the memory clinic. This meeting was the first time I had been able to talk freely about how I felt about anything in front of a mental health professional that was part of the system. The difference for me was that she listened without interrupting even though she had her own agenda to get through she allowed me to set the pace of the meeting. When I was finished and Karen had her say only then did she start her own assessment I hated it as most of the time as I knew that I knew the answer but answers did not come. Instead I got more frustrated, this made the questions appear even harder and by the end of the assessment I felt a real failure. The dementia nurse let's call her Bobby then made one of the best comments I had heard up to now when on completion of the assessment remarked "well I guess we now know that something is not right with your memory".

During the assessment we had told Bobby about the many other types of experiences I was having including new voices (Bobby had taken the fact that I was a voice hearer in her stride) glimpses of things that moved too fast for me to pin down, leaving the gas on, forgetting simple things, being tired, disturbed sleep all the time, thrashing about in bed and tremors in my arm and legs. After we had gone through everything that was happening Bobby for the first time talked about Dementia with Lewy Bodies as a possible diagnosis though she was clear that this was a working diagnoses and that she wanted to look at other possibilities and would discuss with people she worked with to see if a referral to a neurologist might give greater clarity to what was happening. With this the meeting ended though and armed with my next appointment we left. I was now in a hurry to get home, as I wanted to research Parkinson's and Dementia with Lewy Bodies and compare what I found with what I was experiencing. The best description of what to look for in Dementia with Lewy Bodies (DLB) I found was the following from Facty Health Symptoms of Dementia with Lewy Bodies.

"People with dementia with Lewy bodies will generally experience at least two of these three core symptoms":
• Dramatic swings between alertness and drowsiness or confusion. These may happen suddenly and unexpectedly, and can last for differing periods of time

- Parkinson's-like symptoms, i.e. difficulty walking or uncontrollable shaking
- Regular vivid visual hallucinations – these can range from pleasant to disturbing.

Sleep disturbances are also very common in patients with DLB. For example, people with DLB may find it difficult to stay awake during the day, but also difficult to fall asleep at night.

All of the above describe what was happening to me though some days it was much worse than others and conversely some days could be much better than others. It was around this time that my GP decided that I was getting to the stage where I could not work and I was given a sick note and told to stay off work for at least two months. Karen and I had a major discussion that was recorded about what she thought as she saw things happening within me (see Karen's epilogue). I knew my current working life was coming to an end but there was no way I was going to vegetate I needed to find things to do so with Karen I made a list of things that I could try to do that would both keep me stimulated and also be useful to our company. In actual fact there were a number of things I could try to do even though most of them would be new to me. The list we made included creating flyers for events, transferring all our books onto create space so that it would be easier for Americans and Canadians to get them, turning all our training packs into books thereby making them accessible to far more people by reducing the price from around one hundred pounds to ten pounds. All of these tasks would be really valuable for us but they came to me with one little problem and that was technology. Technology and I did not get on when I was working at full capacity so I could not imagine being able to complete these tasks with a wonky memory and crap concentration.

My biggest problem in finding a solution was simple I was still an analogue thinker in a digital world. I needed to stop trying to think outside the box get rid of the box and start to think without the constraints that the box was putting me under. In the end the solution was not to use one computer but to use two computers. In other word's I would work in stereo, simple solution, sanity saved (or so I thought until I tried to put it into action).

Why two computers you may ask? The answer makes sense to me and is that even when I am working at full tilt I will forget how to do something on the computer at this point I would have to come out of the work I was doing, Google what I was trying to do, search the results, find the one that I wanted open it, read it, minimize it go back to the work I was doing and restart only to discover that I have forgotten how to do it again so begins a cycle of switching between the two files that becomes in itself confusing.

Because I have two computers it means that one computer it's always on the piece of work I'm doing whilst the other is normally on You Tube with instructions on how I can do the piece of work. This is brilliant and that it means I save a lot of time going back and forward from file to file. As my memory has got worse this way of working has allowed me to continue at a good pace, this gives me a lot of hope of being able to work for a long time into the future. I am also now using Dragon Dictate to write with, this takes away the need for me to use a key-board as I quite often get confused about where the letters are and often create some amazing looking words that are meaningless. The other reason that not having to use a keyboard is helpful is that one of my medications makes joints and my fingers really sore.

Technology then can be used in a positive way to keep me occupied in a meaningful sense. As a result of technology I have been able to fulfil many of the tasks laid out above, I have also grown in confidence with each success in my new working role. (More about technology later)

I must admit there are still times when I would like to just wallow in self-pity especially when I am trying to do a task and for some reason it is not coming together this is when the rules laid out in part one of this book are really important to me. Having found a way to overcome my analogue way of thinking and becoming what I'd like to term a digital thinker I was feeling quite pleased with myself. I also find it safe to work on my and alone in my office with no one else allowed, so they do not see me especially my family when things do go wrong. When you think of yourself as a person with a cognitive memory problem heading towards the dementia diagnosis there is a lot of shame and guilt that is difficult to talk about. Equally it is difficult for my family to talk to me about what's happening they often find themselves responding to my behaviours or the mistakes that I make. This sometimes leads to strained relationships within our house understanding this means that rule number one for families must be "KEEP TALKING". Part three of this book will deal with the use of technology in more detail.

It was now December 2017 five months since I've seen the psychiatrist and three months had passed since I first saw the dementia nurse and it was coming to the time when I was due to see her again (at the memory clinic). Once again Karen and I headed to the doctor's surgery and once again we waited for a short time before Bobby came into the waiting room and asked us to join her (by now we thought of Bobby as the memory clinic) in the consulting room.

Once the pleasantries were over Bobby went through a number of options they were: Dementia with Lewy Bodies, some other type of neurological problem or perhaps she suggested my problems were a result of stress. This idea intrigued me so I asked her why she thought it might be about stress. This led to a\]wide ranging conversation about stress and that after 20 years of working for myself, stress was something I lived with comfortably therefore we did not see it as the contributing factor. We then went on to talk about what was happening in the here and now and how family members had noticed a worsening of my memory and a greater tendency to fall. Karen talked about the difficulty I was having in terms of sleep especially trying to get to sleep. Bobby told us that she would arrange an appointment with the neurologist and that in the meantime Dementia with Lewy Bodies would remain as the working diagnoses until other neurological causes were ruled out. Seven months later I am still waiting to see a neurologist, and as of yet I have still not even received an appointment. So I have to wait and nothing can be done until that appointment happens

In part three of this book I will bring readers up to date starting from the 31st December 2017. I will also explore the beginnings of my virtual memory or as I prefer to call it plan B.

Part three

The long wait

Chapter Six

It is 3.22am on the 31st of December 2017 the last day of this year is creeping towards daybreak. Sleep is still hard to find and often like tonight I find myself down stairs in the kitchen staring out of our window watching the lighthouse light flash past every few seconds I come too but remain staring mesmerised by the light as it dances dramatically over the ocean before disappearing out of sight for that brief moment before returning. My memory is good at holding recent events for all of 38 hours. Can't sleep so I decide to do what was becoming an ever more regular thing which was to write some of my thoughts about the last day or so before they like the light disappear but unlike the light they will not come back.

Yesterday was a day and a half, I talked to a client who is doing really well as they learn to take more and more control over the voices that constantly corrupt the quality of their life with foul language and innuendo. Karen has also been talking to clients and celebrating with them as they come to realisations in their lives that is allowing them to reconnect with who they are yet we both feel helpless as we watch one of our kids whom we love so much struggle with their sadness; no their grief at a relationship ended.

The cynic, or perhaps even realist within me operates at a shit happens they will get over it level whilst the father part of me just wants to take them in my arms and let that pain dissolve through their tears that need to be released which in my perfect world of my inner dad would heal their heart whilst soaking my shirt.

As I go back upstairs with a fresh cup of tea, my thoughts once again turn to yesterday and in a moment of clarity I remember the whole day as if it was being replayed in holovision right in front of my eyes. (holovision would be my ideal it is essentially 3D television but in the middle of the room not on a wall only in science fiction at the moment) One minute I see Karen coming up stairs with tea and my breakfast of Yogurt, fruit and seeds, the next it is scary daughter (our youngest kid) running into our room and jumping onto our bed to get a cuddle and tell us that she loves us. Scary Daughter is nearly 15 and this is my latest name for her as she changes from girl to woman. It is also true she is scary, one minute she is the ultimate in sweetness and light and in the next she can be a screaming banshee. But not this morning today she is sweetness and light and is talking to us about her exams that are coming up soon.

Next thing I know I am watching myself on the computer I am working on getting all our book titles onto Create Space which is a bit technical so I am using my two computers at once trick. This is where I work on our computer in our (my but don't tell Karen)) study and have my laptop on the desk also in front of me on YouTube so that when I forget what I have to do next I can watch the guide I use in order to get it done properly (who said men can't multitask). Since my memory loss started I have learnt a number of tricks to keep on top of stuff. By that I mean finding and using ways of doing things that means people don't notice my memory problems, more of this later.

I spend a lot of time on the computers now, mainly because people leave me pretty much alone when I am in the study and this means I do not need to pretend I am fully in the same space as people as I have to do when I am in the same room. I find myself having to pretend to be there more and more or alternatively spend a lot more energy in forcing myself to concentrate in situations that have no real meaning to me. Real meaning now there is a thought what is real meaning? The answer to this question is complex as things that had real meaning to me two or even one year ago hold very little meaning to me now and vice-versa.

I must confess that throughout my life I have never known my priorities to change so quickly and radically as they have done since I was given my dementia diagnoses. You would think by now it was time to try to get some sleep but no! for me it was time to choose, time to stop talking and to start doing, time to decide my own future, time to create a plan that I could implement, it was time to make my virtual memory a reality. I spent the rest of the early hours writing how I would go about creating the prototype for my virtual memory that alongside working with my voices both internal and external would be my response to my diagnoses. The result of these early hours can be found below. New-years' eve 2017 was my independence day 2018 would be my year no matter what happened. This was to be the year of memory.

Virtual Memory
Creating A Prototype
December 31, 2017
Overview
Project Background and Description

Having recently received a dementia with Lewy Bodies working diagnosis it became clear to me that the memory loss frightened me more than anything else. My greatest fears in this area were:
1 Forgetting who my family are
2 Forgetting who my wife is
3 Forgetting who I am
These very real fears demand a very real response and with the developments in neuroplasticity and our greater understanding of the role that internal dialogues and both internal and external narratives play in developing our continued sense of who we are it has occurred to Karen and I that we could use what we have learned in working with psychosis to facilitate a new narrative approach to memory that will enable the repositioning of memory through an educational framework by using technology to stimulate neuroplasticity healing activity..

Project Scope
The project is deliberately broad in its scope in order to allow for maximum flexibility during the developmental phase. The scope of the project will include:
  a) A relevant literature review on creation of memory, neuroplasticity in changing neural pathways in brain injury, the use of internal and external dialogues, retention of memory.
  b) Critical memories listing events dates
  c) Who are you? Family, friends, self and others

d) The virtual memory box
e) Using film, audio, pictures and objects to create trigger responses for memory.
f) Developing dialogues for pathway change
g) Mapping the journey

The above list is not exhaustive and will almost certainly change as we integrate existing knowledge with new learning from the literature review. The use of technology both as a receptacle for information and as a motivator for change will be explored.

High-Level Requirements

In order for the project to be successful it must include the following:

An integrated information structure that allows information sharing and updating to be easily achieved.

Validated methodologies for measuring changes to memory retention, cognitive functioning and narratives.

Hardware and Software that is up to tasks required

Deliverables

The main outcome we are seeking from this project is to evidence either a slowing down, a halt in progression or the reversal of a dementia through the use of either internal or external voice dialogues to relocate or hold memory thereby retaining the subjects' sense of self and surrounds.

Partnerships

David Storm RMN, Karen Taylor RMN, Psychologist? Occupational Therapist? Academic Institution

Affected Business Processes or Systems

There will be the need to find some technical expertise specifically around managing data bases

Specific Exclusions from Scope
None
Implementation Plan
The implementation plan will be developed as and when the literature reviews are completed. The literature reviews should be completed by the end of January with the full implementation plan available in early February.
High-Level Timeline/Schedule
The intention is to work to a tight timeline in order to complete the production of a single virtual memory for the pilot subject by the end of January 2019 The pilot subject is Me.

Chapter Seven

Designing My Virtual Memory
January 2018

That's it, my decision has now been made and I have decided to fight the effects of dementia and I am also going to create my own virtual memory. (the virtual memory I want as a back-up plan and as an aid.) Since getting the working diagnoses of Dementia with Lewy Bodies I have been tinkering around with the concepts of virtual memory and how to use teachers voice as an internal way of holding memory whilst the virtual memory will hold memory in an external format.

I have always been interested in memory since reading Steven Rose the making of memory many years ago. Though much has happened in the area of Neuroscience over the resulting years it was this book that helped me understand the dialectical concepts both within politics and society and more importantly it was the beginning of my education around developing ideas of mind body dualism. In order to design a virtual memory, I had to define the border between my own memory and my virtual memory. In doing this I decided that for me the main difference would be that my memories would hold emotion related to the memory whilst my virtual memory would hold information devoid of independent emotion. Any emotion generated would come from my response to the information received from the AI.

I stated earlier that my virtual memory was to be my back up plan and that using neuroplasticity to change my condition was plan A. It seems sensible however to put plan B into development whilst working on plan A. So having made this decision it was now the time to lay out what I am going to need in detail to create the virtual memory. The first thing I needed was a planning method, and it seemed to me that essential lifestyle planning would be the planning tool that would meet my future needs. I guess this begs the question What is essential lifestyle planning?

The following is a short description of essential lifestyle planning that will hopefully give the reader some understanding of the process.

An Overview of
Essential Lifestyle Planning

Adapted from an article by Michael Smull and Susan Burke Harrison
Essential lifestyle planning is a guided process for learning how someone wants to live and for developing a plan to help make it happen. It's also:

- a snapshot of how someone wants to live today, serving as a blueprint for how to support someone tomorrow;
- a way of organizing and communicating what is important to an individual in "user friendly", plain language;
- a flexible process that can be used in combination with other person centered planning techniques; and,
- a way of making sure that the person is heard, regardless of the severity of his or her disability.

Essential lifestyle plans are developed through a process of asking and listening. The best essential lifestyle plans reflect the balances between competing desires, needs, choice and safety.

Developing plans that really reflect how people want to live require:

- The perspectives of those who know and care about the person;
- Their stories about good days and bad; and,
- What they like and admire about the person.

Good plans reflect the perceptions of the focus person and those who know and care about him or her. Learning how people want to live• is children through is you you think I have just the beginning, the foundation. Helping people have their own lives requires changing:

- How we think;
- How we are organized; and
- How we act.

This• then you will are you are here you want to is the process that is now at the center of how I live my life an individualized person centered process geared to helping me retain as much autonomy as possible. As part of this I mapped out all of the things that are essential to me on a daily basis starting from the moment I wake up until my time of going to sleep. It sounds easy enough but when you start to write down everything you do in a day that is essential for your wellbeing the list grows and then grows some more.

My current list (April 2018) is broken down into 8 sections these are:

1) Wake Up

2) Morning
3) Lunch
4) Afternoon
5) Late Afternoon
6) Dinner
7) Evening
8) Bedtime Routine

These sections are just the Essentials for when Karen is not around and when she is around my daily essentials may change. This is also true for weekends and holidays. My planning system must therefore be flexible enough to adapt to an ever changing me and yet keep me on track in being able to maintain control in my life.   An example of this subtle difference between essential and desirable can be when I eat breakfast, the essential is that I eat, the desirable is what I eat.

My future Essentials plan will look something like this:
Monday
Wake Up.

Alexa Alarm 7.00am Alarm goes off and heavy metal music plays this is to ensure that I respond to my alarm and wake up. I then instruct Alexa to tune into radio 4fm to listen to thought for the day. I will also get the latest news briefing from the BBC via Alexa. At 8.15am I will get a reminder from Alexa about having a shower then I will go have a shower, the shower will also be operated by Alexa in terms of controlling temperature thereby ensuring my safety Alexa will also be able to control turning water on and off both via voice control and by use of a reminder Timer.

Morning

Once dressed my Morning begins with breakfast this is normally fresh fruit and Yogurt with a strong cup of tea. After breakfast my day really begins and at 9.30 until 10.15 I do some brain training using my kindle. This is part of my neuroplacisity effort and involves finding five letter words in a set of seven or eight letters. This helps get my brain going in the morning but also makes me use parts of my brain involved in short term memory retention. After brain training it is time to go to my house office and start work normally dealing with e-mails, checking facebook, and other social networks and posting things as required. At 12 Noon Monday, Tuesday, Thursday and Friday I stop to watch the Daily Politics stopping half an hour earlier on Wednesday as it begins at 11.30am.

Lunch
Lunch for me starts at 1 o'clock after I have watched my political program, I like to vary my lunch though I am partial to salmon sweet-corn and mayonnaise I also like soup in the winter though I do get embarrassed when I end up wearing the Soup. I do not mind eating lunch with my family but I am not so good when eating lunch with people I do not know so well. I also take my medication before Lunch finishes at 2 PM and it is time for me to go back to work.

Afternoon
I am normally much better than the afternoon so I tend to do work that requires more concentration or needs me to think more about what I'm doing. I also want to spend at the least one hour in the afternoon writing my journal so I can keep my•
writing are whether it a year are very easily and ACF printer in

the settled fellow already is the all the your options for the are desirous more studies wireless destiny of the up-to-date. I am also happy to do Skype calls in the afternoon. At around 4:30 PM during the school week I need to spend time with my youngest daughter when she comes home from school so we can keep in touch with what is happening in each other's lives. This will also stop me from isolating myself in my study room as this is something I am liable to do if I do not have other things in place to stop me. I also enjoy tea and a biscuit (or two) at around 3.30 PM though the biscuit is not an essential everyday

Late Afternoon

Late Afternoon is the one part of the day that can change a lot depending on what is happening both in my life and in the lives of the rest of the family. At this point of the day I do like to catch up on what is happening in the world hence radio 4 is always on in my office. This would be a normal time for me to call my mom and also my sister.

Dinner

Dinnertime is a family time and we all eat together around the table television is switched off and we use this time as a chance to catch up with each other. We tend to eat very healthy meals particularly we eat vegetarian at least three times a week. Karen drives this healthy lifestyle and she often faces protest from the two children and myself about the meals we are given. Sometimes it might appear that we protest too much as we always eat the food in front of us. It is important that I do eat healthily as it is clear that good nutrition is important when dealing with memory loss. I also take my evening medication at dinner time

Evening

I often refer to the best way of living our lives as living a Mars bar day the reason for this is simple we need to learn to work rest and play. Eight hours a day of work leaves us 16 hours to rest and play getting this balance right is essential to ensure the well-being. Play is something I find difficult mainly because I am too competitive to play games play also requires social interaction and this is something that I do find. Therefore it is really important that I'd take time play in the evening, indeed I would go as far as to say that play for me is an essential part of my life whether I wish to play or not. I may also in the evening do one or two Skype calls with people from other continents. This should however never exceed three calls in any one evening.

Bedtime routine

I guess the most important part of the day for me has to be my bedtime routine. The first thing I do as I prepared for bed is to take my final medications of the day I then get a hot drink taken upstairs to my bedroom and down more often than not go for a bath two relax my muscles especially in my legs. This is important as it helps me to stop thrashing about in the bed this not only helps me but it also helps Karen who suffers a lot if I do not prepare properly. Along with my medications I also take magnesium as part of my bedtime routine. At my bedside I keep the following spray for angina, paracetamol for pain, a cold drink and my kindle in case I cannot get to sleep. I also use the Kindle as a light if I have to get up through the night. Having done all this I can now jump into bed and try to get some sleep.

This way of planning takes up a lot of time in the first instance what you have read up to now is only my routine for one day and in order to create a plan that would honor my routine I would write up my essential routine over the period of one month. This would then give me a smorgasbord of things that I could do every day. In other words I would create a weekly plan to ensure diversity in my life. I have always thought that surprises were an important part of our lives so building surprises into the plan is really important.

Understanding a person's story or narrative is also essential if we are to get the planning process to work properly. This meant that I would have to work with my whole team in an open and honest way therefore I would have to learn to trust them very quickly. This will always be difficult to achieve for me, as one of the things I have noticed is my tendency to become paranoid very easily. Though my paranoia has its roots in things that have happened and I know this, I still have great difficulty in bringing this under control and as a consequence I often find myself losing my temper when I feel paranoid. Being aware of these things has many drawbacks the main one being you know when not to speak to people as well as when you should speak to people. How we hear a person's narrative is also important and we should ensure that we do not rush this process. I am a natural storyteller and so when I tell my story I wish to tell it as a storyteller this again is something I must consider when it comes to telling my team.

Person Centered Planning is not an easy way to work and it is fraught with pitfalls but it is also filled with opportunities and if we are going to change the way people with memory loss are treated in our society then we must start by changing the way we plan. This is how I intend to have my life mapped out as I face what the wheel of time has set before me. Personally I am not yet ready for a formal and detailed essential life plan so what the above plan contains is the bare bones of my plan that will in time be fleshed out and turned into a plan that can be implemented on a daily basis.

The major challenge in this type of planning centers around how we deal with the significant others in a person is life. For myself it would be how can we ensure that Karen's needs are met whilst at the same time keeping me in the centre of the process. There is no easy answer to this and therefore we must rely on our ability to negotiate, whilst making sure that we honor the process. Another challenge when planning especially where they may be some differences in what the people are asking for is to ensure that we hear from as many people as possible who are involved directly in providing services to the person. This should also involve people who are providing non-paid services as well as those we were recompensed for their time. I am sure that this will be an area of discussion that we will come back to as my journey continues.

Conclusion

I should mention that there are other person centred tools that can be used to help a person plan tools such as PATH (planning alternative tomorrows with hope) is one such tool that we would recommend. The main thing of course is that the person at the centre of the planning process is in charge of which tool or tools are used. In chapter 8 I will explore both the use of technologies that can be helpful that are also easily available and also my experience with Alexa as I try to train this AI to become my personal assistant thereby really helping me to go forward into the future with confidence. As I continue to write I find that I am more aware of how my life is maybe going to be affected in the future. I am also aware of how my life is being affected in the here and now just last night my wife pointed out to me that I have become more emotional recently as I have developed the book. I have come to the conclusion that she is right and as I continue writing I am much more in touch with who I am.

Chapter Eight

Throughout January 2018 I spent a lot of time making lists of all the things that needed to be done to move my virtual memory forward. The great thing about lists is that they act as a wonderful way to avoid doing the actual work and for much of January this is how I avoided facing what was happening. One of the first things I had to recognize was that I no longer did much work outside of my office and creating lists was one of the ways I tried to justify my existence. It was so bad that I was beginning to make lists of lists a sign that I was losing the plot. When you realize that some of the things you are doing are meaningless you must either, change what you're doing and then get on with the task in hand or you change nothing and vegetate.

Feeling down is something most people who have had a diagnosis of memory loss or dementia seem to get regularly. This feeling that some may call depression would hit me every four weeks or so and would last between a day and a week. It seemed to me that in the first months of 2018 I was afflicted with my own personal black dog that hit me with low moods, lots of doubts and an eating away of my confidence. What if I'm wrong I would often think and I find myself condemned to a life of ever decreasing memories what then would I have to look forward to. It comes as a shock when I realize that if the worst were to happen then I wouldn't care probably because I would not know it was happening. For almost 3 months this became my thinking pattern, I called it stinking thinking. It was very clear that if I did not change my thinking I would become stuck in what Karen and I called the illness to trap.

This would leave me into a never-ending circle of despair. It's worth noting that even after years of successfully working with other people when it came to working with myself I got stuck.

Stinking thinking is for me the greatest challenge that faces our society today when we are dealing with dementia or memory loss. It is endemic within the professions that treat us without compassion and this is passed on to our families when they are told it is a degenerative progressive illness for which there is no cure in other words the beginning of our post diagnoses is geared to accepting that the next real stop is death. There are innovative projects happening within the UK but their impact is minimal especially when austerity driven budgets encourage systems to work to the lowest common denominator. It appears to me that that the only time politicians care about us is when we are in work, between 18 and 65 and in good health. Stepping outside of these parameters makes you a burden on the rest of our community in the eyes of many of our political leaders throughout the world. This is especially true when it comes to conditions like dementia (one of the so called no hope conditions) this is the type of things that I spend too much time thinking about and I end up doing little whilst this fear of being a burden dominates my thoughts. Even my wife Karen has her moments of doubt about her ability to see this journey through to the end if it starts to go badly. As time has gone on I have found it easier to talk about these things. Talking without action is paramount to waiting for God so for the rest of this chapter I am going to talk about actions. One of our children is technology mad and as soon as he could he bought himself and Amazon Echo so it was no longer a matter of talking about using a virtual assistant I was at last able to see how it might work. It did not take me long to be convinced that I needed my own so very quickly I thought, and within days I had an Amazon Show. The Amazon Show is the latest in the range of virtual assistants the main difference from the Amazon Echo is that the Show Has a screen that allows you to watch things as well this hear. When my virtual assistant arrived I was the happiest man alive until of course I tried to get the virtual assistant to understand what I was saying in my fine Scottish accent. I would say to her put on radio four and she would reply "I don't know that one" I tried everything including speaking very slowly. This seemed only to confuse her more and I found that I had to make my accent less thick. The other thing that was difficult was stopping my children from getting her to do silly things like telling jokes or even worse getting her to say things like I love you.

Once we got over the language barriers I started to explore what we could actually do together I was able to set reminders for times to take medication, appointments at the hospital, going to see my GP and when to meet friends in town. I was also able to set alarms to get up in the morning or to tell me when something I was cooking was ready. These simple things increased my self-confidence and allowed me to tackle things I was frightened I would lose. Alexa (that is the name of my virtual assistant) had in my opinion proven her worth and I set about planning how I would use that technology to maintain my independence and ensure that my family felt that I was safe.

Safety is one of the issues that can sometimes consume much of our loved one's time. My youngest daughter would often shout to me to ask if I was all right because she feared for my safety. I had to learn that this was her fear and she had the right to have this fear I got used to saying I'm okay. I recall one time when I was away with Karen just after the recovery camp we went to a shopping centre in Shrewsbury, we went our own ways in the centre and agreed to meet each other at the stairs that led to the car park. I walked around the centre and very quickly found myself turned around and hopelessly lost. No matter how hard I tried I could not find my way to the stairs. I could feel myself panic and for the first time in many years I felt totally out of control. It did not occur to me to ask someone for directions I just kept walking looking for the way out and in my failure I became more and more anxious. Eventually I find a way out of the centre and decided to wait outside. I knew that Karen would be looking for me and 15 minutes later she found me.

I guess this was the point in our lives where what was happening to me became much more real it was also the first time that I had felt unsafe and the cause of my feeling was my condition. The irony of this story was that the shopping centre I was in was designated a dementia friendly area I just had not asked for help. So for me it is no longer a matter of if at first you don't succeed try and try again it has now become if at first you don't succeed then ask for help. Asking for help is often difficult because it does make you vulnerable, as you are aware that your independence is beginning to disappear. One of the things I learned in mental health was the need to explore the issue of independence against the reality of Inter-dependence. I realized that this was something I was going to have to relearn and more importantly apply to my own life. I also made a note to find a technological solution to getting lost. At this time if you went into my office you would find post-it notes all over the place with sheets of paper with scribbled notes reminding me of things I had to do. I had not yet come to the realization that I needed to organize a lot more of my life than I had in the past. Indeed I now knew that I would have to move away from my chaotic nature to one that was almost over ordered. I guess it was at this moment I realized that what was needed would be an integration of brain power and computer memory in such a way that the outcome would let me remain well at least appear to remain in control of my life.

Without any manipulation on my part I am about to return to where I started in this chapter and that is in order to move forward I need to start by making yet another list. In chapter six I laid out the components of my essential lifestyle plan yet if you explore this plan you can see very quickly that it really pertains to the maintenance of my working life. In other words even though an essential lifestyle plan is detailed it is not detailed enough to meet my real needs. The reason for this is simple; time or should I say not enough time I spent around an hour working on my plan yet it covers a very small part of my life indeed the reality is that the plan only takes into account one day of a year that is three hundred and sixty five days long. With the best will in the world we cannot plan every second of our lives and although we talk about flexibility we are very inflexible in how we live our lives.

I remember once many years ago the organization I was then a member of wrote to Prince Charles to ask him if he would come to our conference and make a presentation. To our surprise we received a reply that told us we had made it through that first of a series of diary meetings and that the Palace would be in touch with us at a future date to tell us whether the Prince would be able to attend or not. In the end he did not attend. The purpose of this story is to show that planning is not is a linear process but is multi-faceted and that planning often needs to be changed to meet changing needs. It was with this in mind that I decided to call a meeting with Karen to begin to create a diary for the next three months.

All the information that we would gather at this meeting would be fed into my virtual memory and the result would be a calendar around which I could build what I wanted to do and achieve over that three months it is my intention to have this meeting tomorrow and then I will write up the process though I promise not to bore you with the content of the meeting. One of the hardest things to get happening in my life is to get Karen to attend planning meetings of any kind, especially ones that I call. So it was no surprise to me when my first attempt at getting a meeting was met with "not at the minute love I'm busy" not to be deterred I then moved to plan two which involves enticing Karen to come out and have a coffee whilst we are in town (we have to go into town anyway) Karen responds by suggesting I get the bus into town on my own because it will save on the use of fuel. I do sometimes think that Karen is deaf to what I say when I am not speaking or perhaps I am once again not telling Karen what I actually need perhaps it will be third time lucky.

So it was with slight trepidation that I once again approached Karen and to be honest we agreed a compromise that involved me going to town on the bus (on my own) then Karen joining me in town in the late afternoon so we could have our planning meeting before going to a concert later that evening. Going into town on my own has become a bit of a long haul journey for me, as there is so much preparation involved in getting myself ready and willing to make the trip. This requires me to make notes of what I am going into town to do. I will put this information into both paper and digital formats to ensure that I get all I want to do done. I then have to make sure I have my wallet, bus pass, notebook, kindle and my coat before going out to get the bus. Although all of this seems simple enough I find myself running around like the well-known blue assed fly and as the time for the bus gets closer I once again go online to check the bus time and discover to my horror that although there is a 12.40pm bus it only runs on a Saturday and since this is Tuesday the next bus is not until 1.50pm far too late to get me into town for my hospital appointment. Gingerly I approach Karen and tell her that there is no bus at 12.40pm to which she simply replies I will take you in and we can start our meeting in the car. So after all the hassle we had gone back to plan A.

The car journey takes around 40 minutes and so it did give us time to have our meeting but as usual we got sidetracked and it was not until late afternoon that we got around to having our "meeting". As meetings go this one was not bad Karen only checked her social media and emails four times, she has somehow managed to affect this way of sitting with you and making you think she is giving you her undivided attention. This only falls apart when you sit and wait for her reply to something you ask her you wait, you wait and you wait and then she will speak and normally she says' "What do you think?" She is looking for me to answer and use my answer to give her some clues to what I was talking about, this way she will save face and be able to respond in an appropriate way to whatever I have been talking about for the last twenty minutes or so. I have two options at this point the first is to call her out and insist that she answers first; a tactic that is fraught with dangers' if you want my honest opinion. Or I could go with the second option which is to just concede gracefully and tell her what I think at the same time feeling as I have given her a get out of jail free card. I of course decide option two is the better choice it also means I will not be subjected to the Karen glare, a famously foul look that she has perfected.

Essentially we decided what my next three months covering June, July and August of 2018 would look like so that I could build in the things I needed to do to enable me to do some work on myself. We also decided that after this year I was not doing any more training tours a major decision for us and one that I will no doubt fret about for some considerable time. It is difficult for me to imagine not working with people around both the UK and further afield. So my first instinct was to kick back against this decision seconds after we had made it, the truth however was that although my mind was willing my body was no longer up to the task. This did not mean that I would never go away just that when I did it would be for shorter periods and probably in the UK. Even if I did occasionally go overseas I would let Karen do the work and take a bit of a holiday for myself. Indeed even in the next month I am in France for a week and in England for two weeks and on the island for ten weeks this is a reversal of what my life was; then I would normally be away for ten weeks and at home for three weeks. If I am to take my own health seriously then I guess that the new balance is just about right for surely I would be able to do a lot of work on myself in a ten week period. This new work life balance does not leave me feeling happy, rather it tells me that I am making myself a priority at last. As you can see much is changing in my life and my family and I have to adapt to these changes. This is a time when we also have to face our demons. As stated earlier in the book my fear is not being able to recognize my children or my partner or perhaps even myself. At this stage I would be afraid that I could no longer make decisions that were based on any rationality.

In the next chapter we will explore the issue of capacity focusing on how we might prepare for such an event, not in a negative way but in a way that preserves our autonomy and retains our dignity.

Chapter Nine

The question of capacity is something that those suffering memory loss or dementia will sooner or later have to face up to and this was the same for me. In many ways you can laugh off occasionally or even more frequently leaving the gas or electricity or putting your shirt on the wrong way round but when it comes to giving your bank details even online to a legal company that allows them to start taking money from your account for something you do not want then perhaps you need to explore whether your capacity is up to the task. Even worse I could not remember that I had done this luckily the company involved immediately refunded the money I spent.

The hardest thing about this is not having the conversation about what has happened it is about coming to terms with the consequences of your actions. Having dementia does not make you stupid and deep down you know what must be done but giving up control of your own money and the decisions you can make because you have this control is an agonizing move as you can see yourself losing your autonomy. But what we must also understand is that it is equally difficult for family members to take this control away. It is incumbent on us then to begin these difficult conversations well in advance of actions having to be taken. In many ways I was lucky I never really had anything to do with the money from the house as Karen was in control of our budgets. This meant that most of the changes for me were nothing more than cosmetic although I had to give up my business credit card.

Although I never said anything at the time this was another lesson in Interdependence.

Giving up control of money was only the start of the process off understanding what lack of capacity could mean. Recently I decided I needed to protect my family further I also needed to protect myself. In order to do this Karen and I went to see our solicitor. The reason for the visit was simple we wanted him to draw up a power of attorney so that Karen would have wide ranging decision making powers on my behalf.

I did not realize how wide ranging these powers would be until I sat with the letter from the solicitor in my hand: I read the first paragraph:

General Powers
"My Attorney may manage my whole affairs as my Attorney thinks fit and shall have full power for me and in my name or in her own name as my Attorney to do everything regarding my estate which I could do for myself and that without limitation by reason of anything contained in this power of attorney or otherwise"

"What is this" I asked myself as I looked at the second paragraph:

Welfare Powers
"In the event of my being incapable in terms of the act to make decisions about my personal welfare, then my Attorney may make decisions on my behalf in relation to my personal welfare in their capacity as my welfare Attorney. I have considered how my incapacity will be determined".

Two paragraphs and it might have looked like I had signed my life away though nothing could be further from the truth as far as I was concerned. The reality for me was that I had ensured that those I trusted most would if and when the time came be able to protect me by making decisions on my behalf that they knew would be in line with my wishes. There is an important point here in that it would be easy to put off this type of decision thinking that there was plenty time to get around to dealing with it. My reasoning tells me that there is lots of time until it runs out then it is too late and the people who you would have trusted are kept out of the process because of bureaucratic nonsense.

There is never a good time to do this kind of thing but what I am sure of is it needs to be done sooner rather than later. This means that it is necessary to have the conversation as soon as you are aware that there is a problem that may affect your capacity. By doing this we protect our own integrity and that of our families. We are also being proactive in retaining our autonomy. If this all sounds like a contradiction it is probably because that is exactly what it is. Always remember that at the end of the day you do not need to sign, having read my document I have decided that I will sign.

Having signed the papers my financial affairs are now in order and information held about me can now be seen by the people I trust, my family are empowered by that signature to act with my full authority and you know what that makes me feel good. For myself the welfare powers are far more important in that not only can the person consent to treatment on my behalf they can refuse such consent. They can also exercise all rights of access to personal data and records held about me. These welfare powers are important for us as I have decided with my partner at what point I would not want treatment to continue and these powers allow her to keep that in our control. Of course there are bits I don't like things like "to make such decisions relating to my dress, diet and personal appearance as are appropriate" or even worse "to decide with whom I should or should not consort". I mean who in their right mind would allow their partner to dress them ("that would be you" one of my voices just said).

This is where you have to learn to trust like you have never trusted before. This can be difficult especially given that paranoia is a common experience connected to cognitive impairment and dementia. For myself I find checking things out with people helps me keep paranoia at bay, though sometimes the way I speak when I am checking stuff out can lead to arguments that can increase my paranoia so even here it is important to take care in the way I go about doing or saying things.

It would be fair to say that the third section of this book is all about communication and I am finding more and more of my thinking is about how to communicate with the various people both individually and in groups that I am involved with in my social, medical, family, spiritual and work life. Equally how people communicate with me is important, already I have become aware of a group of people in our society that I call the thoughtless you can tell who is part of this group the minute you meet them for they will talk to the person you are with as if you are not there, normally opening with how is Ron doing? This is thoughtless on their part and what makes it worse is the amount of times I do nothing about it letting it happen and in effect I am re-enforcing thoughtlessness's view of the world. I think this is something that we need to work together to change for example I do expect people who are with me to challenge this type of behavior for when they do not I become less of a person and more of an object. It is also up to us who experience memory loss to educate wider society about the disabling effects that society can have on us.

It is all very well communicating about the safe areas of our lives but there are parts of our lives that are very difficult to talk about for example I find talking about intimacy almost impossible, I found it equally difficult before my memory problems now it has become a greater burden that I fear will consume me. This has meant I become less and less intimate with my partner as I cannot talk about my inability to feel intimate it does' appear to me that my sexual identity is being stolen faster than my memory. Probably like many others this inability to talk openly about sex or sexual identity has its roots in my own childhood. As a survivor of childhood sexual abuse I need to find ways of protecting myself from those memories in case they become disconnected from me as a person. This possible disconnect was brought to my attention by David Storm the director of aged care services in Cumbria.

David (a psychiatric nurse by background) is one of the most innovative people involved in the delivery of services to elderly people both with functional illnesses or dementia. He noticed that many elderly people who were hearing voices and had a dementia the voices in many cases could be linked to the clients lived experience. In response to this realization CD set up hearing voices groups for elderly people regardless of whether their diagnosis was one of dementia or some form of functional illness. The importance of what David has done did not mean anything to me until I myself started suffering from memory loss it is much easier for me now to envisage for example hearing the voice of the catholic priest saying "it is your fault you lead me on you deserve to burn in hell" and because the event can no longer be remembered I believe it would be easy for me to respond to this in a very negative way. This makes it much more important that when these things are happening we can fall back to a clear narrative that helps all understand what is happening.

Conclusion

In conclusion I would argue that bringing together narrative, technological and neuroplasticity approaches will give many of us the opportunity to reclaim our lives. We must not forget three other areas of our lives that need to be addressed these are: our spiritual well-being, our physical well-being and last but not least our nutritional well-being. These will be explored in the final chapter of this book.
Chapter Ten

In chapter four readers were introduced to some of the terms used in narrative ways of working. In this chapter we will build on our understanding of narrative work by exploring how narrative working might be used in conjunction with neuroplasticity to help both my family and I deal differently with our possible futures. A grouping composed of mainly social workers that were rooted in systemic family therapy developed narrative therapy. Much of the development of this approach has come from both the writings and practice of Michael White and David Epston. The central tenant of narrative work is that "the person is not the problem, the problem is the problem" (O'Hanlon 1994). The person is seen as being different from the problem, but in a relationship with the problem this separation is achieved through a process called externalization by which a person can step back and examine their relationship with the problem. For Example: If I externalize (separate) my memory loss from myself I can then ask the following question to myself "How is memory loss controlling my life?" thereby the problem is now being seen as something that is affecting the person rather than being part of the person. O'Hanlon (1994) sets out seven steps within the narrative approach these are:

1. **Collaborate with the person or the family in coming up with a mutually acceptable name for the problem.** Applying this to my own situation the name for my problem would be dementia.
2. **Personify the problem and attribute oppressive intentions and tactics to it.** The problem (dementia) is trying to disrupt my family life by creating division in the family. It also does things that make both family members and I fearful.
3. **Investigate how the problem has been disruptive, dominating, or discouraging the person or the family.** There are times when dementia can make members of my family fear for my safety it can leave the gas on or not turn the water off. There is also times when I feel dementia has shamed me and so I can easily let dementia convince me to stay away from people and I will quickly become isolated and down.
4. **Discover moments when the client hasn't been dominated or discouraged by the problem or his/her life has not been disrupted by the problem.** There are days when dementia seems less active than others and then I feel much better. Before

dementia came along I felt in control of all parts of my life. My family was also in a much better place before dementia interfered with our family life.

5. **Find historical evidence to bolster a new view of the person as competent enough to have stood up to, defeated or escaped from the dominance or oppression of the problem.** My family and friends have reminded me that I have overcome a similar experience in the past with a problem that was called schizophrenia

6. **Evoke speculation from the person and the family about what kind of future is to be expected from the strong, competent person that has emerged.** I can live my life not my label Living is something I choose while a label is something chosen by a professional.

7. **Find or create an audience for perceiving the new identity and new story.** The audience for my new story will be those who read this book and those who then hear my new story. Part of this will involve exploring the identity of dementia further.

It is possible to apply the above steps to any issue and with anyone; Michael White stated that there are a number of benefits that flow from using a narrative approach.

Possible benefits of narrative ways of working Include:

1. Decreases unproductive conflict between people, including disputes over who is responsible for the problem.

2. Undermines the sense of failure that has developed for many people in response to the continuing existence of the problem despite their attempts to resolve it.

3. Paves the way for people to cooperate with each other, to unite in a struggle against the problem and to escape its influence in their lives.

4. Opens up new possibilities for people to take action to get

back their lives and relationships from the problem and its influence.
5. Frees people to take a lighter, more effective and less stressed approach to serious problems.
6. Presents options for dialogue about the problem.

These six benefits would all be positive for people with memory problems' their friends and family as they are all areas of almost daily concern for us. I know that unproductive conflict is a common result of dementia and can do so much damage not only to me but also to the ones I love. Like many I also find it all too easy to feel a failure and that feeling if taken fully on board can both overwhelm and disable me and then impact negatively on my family. When we work together as a family unit we achieve far greater outcomes than when we remain stuck in our silos. As a family we enjoy laughter far more than the miseries that can (if we give them a chance) take over our lives. Even using these techniques on their own changes our lives. The conversation can change from doom and gloom to opportunity and hope, from negative to positive, from hate to love, from glass half empty to glass half full, from victim to victor and most importantly from dementia to Ron. This is how I see the conversations I will be having with the people around me and by doing this together with neuroplasticity techniques to change pathways in my brain I do expect that at some point I will be able to first stop the decline, then consolidate and then reverse what has happened by letting my brain change itself. I am well aware that making this type of statement will be seen as creating false hope. Scientists and clinicians have long believed and many still do that a damaged or an aging brain is unable to repair, reorganize, or regenerate under any circumstances. Brain development was considered to occur during our very early development, with little or no ability for neuronal tissue to change with injury, aging or training.

However, the last decades of neuroscience research paint a radically different picture of the brain's ability to change its structure and function. It is now widely believed that new neurons and synapses are generated throughout life and neural pathways continually remodel in response to changes in the organism's internal and external environment. Although these phenomena appear to be more pronounced during early development, research suggests the brain maintains its ability to change its structure and function throughout life and well into old age.

Evidence suggests that older adults have been shown to utilize additional or altogether different brain areas, presumably as a compensatory mechanism for age-related cognitive decline, and may employ unique strategies for storing and recalling information as they age. The extent to which these capabilities are maintained in the presence of dementia pathology holds important implications for developing evidence-based interventions. The ability of the brain to change its architecture and function is referred to broadly as *plasticity*. Plasticity implies a degree of malleability; brain organization is altered during the course of maturation, adaptation to environmental changes, or post-injury compensation. The mechanisms of plasticity are plentiful and include neurogenesis, (This is the process by which new neurons are formed in the brain) synaptogenesis, (This is the formation of synapses between neurons in the nervous system) and angiogenesis, (is the process of creating new blood vessels from pre-existing blood vessels. The process is vital for the growth and development of an organism) to name but a few.

Changes may occur at the cellular level through adaptation of neurons and supporting cells or through adaptation of dendrites and synapses due to environmental stimuli. In the damaged brain, it is thought that these changes occur in response to the limitations imposed by brain pathology in an attempt to maintain functional ability. Several terms are often used interchangeably in relation to the broad concept of plasticity including neuronal plasticity (or neuroplasticity), brain plasticity, or cognitive plasticity. While neuronal plasticity implies structural modifiability at the synaptic level and brain plasticity refers to alterations in the activation of brain networks, cognitive plasticity refers to the ability of an individual to improve performance after training. More broadly, plasticity herein may be conceptualized as brain adaptation in response to stressors induced by aging or neuropathology. Taking all the information we have gathered from narrative working and neuroplasticity I believe we can put together individualized programs that will enable people like me to regain or retain full cognitive functions. This may well involve creating an image in your mind and within that image holding a memory perhaps in pictorial form attaching that memory to neurons and then firing the neurons from the centre of where short term memory is held into the part of the brain that converts short-term memories into long-term ones. By using visualisation I am hoping to stimulate neurons into creating space in my brain to hold these memories effectively so that I can recall these memories when required. As well is doing this it is my intention to continue doing mind exercises that will strengthen my ability to concentrate. I know that this will take time to achieve and I may not notice anything during the first few months of trying. As I sit here I am thinking it all looks so easy on paper the challenge will be can I maintain this confidence and still hold on to it in two or even five years' time.

Chapter Eleven
The Spiritual, The Physical and The Edible

In this chapter I wish to explore three areas of my life that are becoming more important to me as I go forward in this journey these are my Spiritual life, my Physical life and my Nutritional life. People who know me will be laughing their heads off at the very thought of me talking about one of these areas never mind all three but I will have to handle the laughers as it seems to me that these three areas will become even more important than they are now as I progress on this quest for wellness. I have come to the conclusion that our here industry pays lip service to our spirituality physicality and nutritional lives.

Spirituality

As I was looking at spirituality within dementia it became clear that this area of our lives is in the main glossed over and beyond asking what religion you are (if any) very little appears to be investigated as to your beliefs. In deed in one paper on spirituality and dementia all that was written was that any type of service for people with dementia should be very short as they might start moving around and being disruptive. This makes God sound very dementia unfriendly something that I'm sure that God would not like, the God I believe in would-be dementia friendly john 3v16 states "For God so loved the World that he gave his only son" there is no qualification in this statement that is: it does not say that God loves the people of the world except of course those with dementia because they cannot sit down for long periods or stay quiet for an hour at a stretch. Many years ago someone I knew told me a story that I have always remembered it is about how God views people it goes something like this: in an old monastery some 40 monks lived and worked, they would work all day and then after the evening meal they would gather in the chapel to praise God by singing and meditating on the Bible. By all accounts they were not very good singers but God would sit in heaven and listen to them as their singing came from the heart. Then one day a new monk joined the brothers and sisters he had the voice of an angel and in the evenings when they came to the chapel his voice would rise above the others. One by one the other monks stopped singing until within a matter of weeks he would sing every evening alone whilst the rest of the brothers and sisters listened. One night the Abbot heard a noise coming from the chapel she went to investigate and there in the centre of the chapel stood an archangel of God. The archangel looked down at the Abbot and said "I have been sent by God to ask you why the monks have stopped singing" "We have not stopped singing instead we have a new brother who has a voice so beautiful that he now sings for all of us" replied the Abbot. At that moment the angel disappear and in its place the Abbot felt the presence of God and God spoke saying "I have heard this one voice and though it is pleasing it does not compare to the beauty I hear when you all sing" with this the presence of God left the chapel. The very next morning the Abbot called together all love the brothers and sisters and said "never again shall anyone person be allowed to sing on their own in the chapel, from this day we shall all sing and praise God together". I guess what I am trying to say in telling this story is that we often get caught up in rules of social niceties and even when these rules do not exist we make them up. Even the word spirituality suggests a place in the world that by its very nature must be dementia friendly. It is also clear that there is a great difference between spirituality and religion. So continuing the status quo is not an option and therefore we must offer a smorgasbord of spiritual opportunities and experiences that allow the possibility of growth for people with dementia regardless of prejudicial views about these people in terms of their capacity to take part in spiritual practice. As a believer I feel very strongly that I do indeed stand in the presence of God and that God delights in me as a part of creation whether I have dementia or not. I do not want my spiritual life self-diminished by a system that believes only in itself to the exclusion of other ways of seeing the beauty of the human spirit or soul. Creating dementia friendly ways and places of worship should create an environment of freedom rather than a regimented view of God. Leonard Cohen once said that he had spent a great deal of his life trying to follow the great religions but happiness still kept breaking through to him. It is obvious to me that we need to create dementia friendly spiritual services in line with an already dementia friendly God.

Please Remember Me

If I forget God Does God cease to be,
Or even worse Does God forget me,
Will my sin be forgiven, if I don't know it's sin,
Can it be that dementing will change everything

I thought I would walk in the shadow of death
And never fear any type of Ill,
But when the shadow is a dementia death,
Then I'm pretty sure I will,

If only one prayer I could send,
It really would have to be
If through dementia, I forget you God
Then please remember me

Physical

We often hear "experts" telling us that we need to keep too an exercise program especially as we get older or have conditions such Diabetes, Heart disease, Strokes and dementias what they do not tell us is how to pay for gym membership or how to find the money to buy the equipment for home use. There are a number of reasons within the dementia community that make accessing physical activity at best difficult and at worst impossible. These include declining confidence in our abilities, inappropriately designed residential aged care facilities or risk averse cultures that do not fully understand the real risk of not doing physical exercise that those with dementia face. I am lucky in this regard in that I am (at the time of writing) undergoing an eight-week program within the Gym that is designed to increase my confidence and also to help develop a longer-term plan for my fitness that takes into account my condition. There are only four of us in the exercise group and this means that we are getting the individual attention that I for one need. But physicality does not begin and end with exercise and it is important that this is both acknowledged and explored. It is not my intention to write about physicality in great detail in this book as it is an area that things will change over the next year or two and therefore there will be more in Book Two. (I guess this is a nice way of saying that exercise has not been a priority of mine up till now). We are all aware of their health benefits of exercise in terms of our physical health but neuroscience has attributed far greater benefits to the simplest form of exercise walking. The neuroscientist Anthony Hannan working with others has done a series of experiments that will change our understanding of the role of environment and exercising in altering the course of catastrophic neurodegenerative disorders that were believed to have a genetic basis.

Huntington's disease is a more terrifying degenerative movement disorder than Parkinson's it is a genetic disorder if a parent has it at child has a 50% chance of getting it too usually between the age of 30 and 45 it is currently thought to be incurable. Its victims progressively lose the ability to move normally, they developed severe jerking movements, become depressed then demented, and die a premature death. It enfeebles the part of the brain called the striatum, which is dysfunctional in Parkinson's disease.

The team used young mice that had had the human Huntington's disease gene transplanted into them. Over time the mice developed the disease. The team studied the effects of providing some of the mice with the running wheel whilst other mice were left to their own devices. The mice that were given nothing to exercise on, contracted Huntington's disease as expected whilst those mice that had the wheel to play on also contracted Huntington's onset was delayed by a significant length of time in fact transferring it into human years the life expectancy in the wheel group was ten plus years greater than those mice who get nothing. I acknowledge that it is difficult to extrapolate literally from an animal life span to a human life span. The research team in this instance based their outcomes by using 2 years as the life span of a mouse. This offers us exciting possibilities going forward in planning activities both away from home and at the house. My regime currently includes warm up, bike, weights, treadmill, step ups and of course a warm down. I have had to visit to the gym at the date of writing so I am in no way claiming that working out helps stop or reduce the time we are affected with, cognitive memory problems. At the very least the workout in the gym should over time make me feel better. I find doing exercise in a controlled setting where people are keeping an eye on me much easier than trying to exercise on my own without someone there to motivate me. I am therefore excited about the future and what it holds for me in the area of physicality

Edibility

A great deal has been written recently about the use of food and food nutrition as a way of preventing or even curing dementia. So having read a great deal about how we can use nutrition as a way of dealing with neurodegenerative problems I am reminded of ways that schizophrenia has been treated using fish oils and other nutrients. One book I would recommend is: "The Mind Diet A Scientific Approach to Enhancing Brain Function and Helping Prevent Alzheimer's and Dementia" By Maggie Moon Lays out the facts around the links between poor nutrition, heart disease and/or cognitive decline or dementia in an understandable way. The book talks about the Mediterranean diet the importance of fish and Olive oil feature throughout the 75 recipes in the book, Combining this way of eating with exercise and meditation can create a protective layer of defense that will hold off the insidious assault that is dementias' hallmark approach to taking control over someone's life. I will now spend the next few months trying to put what I have learned into practice on myself.

The Kitchen in My Mind

I went into the kitchen,

For what I do not Know,

The Kitchen though was not there!

So where the hell did it go

It was not outside in the barn,

Nor up our brand new stairs,

It was not near the living room,

I could've sworn I'd seen it there,

So Karen said to me

Tis' where its' always been,

Scary Daughter said to Karen

He is trying not to clean,

He is trying to avoid the dishes

It's very plain to see,

He is Just a lazy Wassock

Tis not his memory

I headed to the kitchen,

With Tail betwixt my legs,

A basket of washing waited me there,

Karen supplied the pegs,

Go and hang the washing out

Upon the washing line,

Then come back and do the dishes,

then you'll have done your time,

Now the moral of this story,

Is there for all to see,

If you cannot find the kitchen,

Do not blame your memory

Part Four
Final Countdown

When a memory disappears
Deep into the nothingness we call time,
Then that memory tries to reappear
In my head because it is mine

Like a soldier sent over the top
It fights the muck and slime
Of all my other troubled thoughts
Caught in this moment of time.

Caught in this moment of time
As if stuck in a revolving door
Caught in this moment of time
Like a shadow on dance floor

I'm always on the move
But never catching mine
For I am trapped, imprisoned
Yes I'm caught in this moment of time

Caught in this moment of time
I look back as tomorrow nears
Caught in this moment of time
As my fear relives my fears
Caught in this moment of time
As yesterday dares to become today,
But now I know this moment of time
I'm no longer condemned to stay

For I will learn to fly
In the nothingness we call time
And I will capture and caress
That memory because it is mine

Without fear I will stare
Into my lived muck and slime,
For I am free, unshackled unfettered
As I walk through that moment in time.

Ron Coleman
March 2018

Epilogue
By Karen Taylor

What is it like to find out that your partner is losing his memory. Two years ago I would have given you an abstract interpretation based on my first 5 years as a registered mental nurse, when I mainly worked with families where Dementia was present.

Now it is a reality for myself and my family.

Firstly, it's insidious, it creeps in, you doubt its existence, you make excuses for it, deny it, do not see it, banish it. This isn't happening, it's something else.
You notice that the person you love is slightly different, but he has just been through a year of trauma, heart attacks, being stuck in Australia away from the family, of course he is going to be different, its depression, its stress, its tiredness.

Back at the beginning of 2017 I was away a lot working in Australia trying to establish a recovery house and other projects, but it was becoming clear this wasn't going to be easy. I returned home in February for a filming project on our work in psychosis, we had a camera crew coming to Lewis and several guests all voice hearers and we were going to spend a week together exploring voices through voice dialogue and sculpting, as well as co- facilitating with Ron, I was cook and taxi driver for the week. First thing I noticed was Ron was incredibly sleepy. He would keep nodding off during the filming and had very little energy. Despite this the week went very well, Ron had also been diagnosed with a sclerotic artery in his neck that was very blocked so he wasn't getting enough oxygen to his brain.

I must admit to feeling very pressured and stressed during the week, as Ron was unable to help very much and didn't seem very "with it" although when awake his facilitating was brilliant. I had to leave pretty soon after back to Australia and returned home again towards the end of March. He was very much inside himself, awaiting an operation in Inverness to unblock his carotid artery, I think he was worried about dying on the operating table which was perfectly reasonable considering what he had been through the year before.

My energy was mainly with the kids as I was away from them a lot. Francesca had noticed that Ron was leaving the cooker on and other odd things but I put it down to the artery problem. I was worrying about whether the operation would happen whilst I was at home, not wanting to be away in Australia, that worry was taken away from me when my visa was denied at the beginning of April, so I was able to go with him to Inverness he had the operation on my birthday.

The Operation was very successful and very quickly the sleepiness subsided, my mind was on how to keep our company going and finding work, but now being at home all the time I could also begin to see that Ron was still struggling with memory but also more worrying he was losing his ability to do arithmetic. I had to take over all the accounts and the VAT, we finally talked it through and went to the doctors and explained what was happening, the doctor did some quick tests and agreed there might be a problem and we were referred to the psychiatrist.

I had no idea how fearful Ron was about going back into psychiatry, I reflect back and realise I was trying so hard to juggle everything that his feelings were probably at the bottom of the pile. But the psychiatrist raised my hackles, he tried to play light of the memory test, I remember arguing with him that he was doing the test with no context to Ron's abilities as an ex accountant with numbers and that it was serious that Ron couldn't subtract 7 from 86 and so on. We left with a diagnosis of mild memory impairment.

I suppose that on one hand I wanted his problems to be seen and understood, on the other hand in day-to-day life I would compensate or dismiss his struggles. We were also struggling with money issues and other seemingly more pressing issues, so I put dementia on the back burner. Its also confusing one day Ron would remember most things others he would be more vacant, I would find myself testing him, is he faking it, all sorts of idea's floated around.

As we progressed to the summer, we both realised the memory problems were not going away so asked the GP to refer Ron to the memory clinic nurse. Ron started looking at ways he could help himself and the film crew came back to do some work with just us around Ron's memory. We were filmed taking about how we felt, bizarrely this was the first time we had a really straight intimate talk about how we were feeling. The plan was for Ron to see if teacher one of his voices would dialogue with me, as he wanted teacher to learn some of his memories and the thought was that if Ron couldn't dialogue with me then teacher could.

We ran the recovery camp in September, it was again stressful for me as I had to do all of the organising, we just managed to break even but the camp was a success, again we had the film crew there and again had our second most intimate chat. This was also about talking about letting me dialogue with teacher, this hadn't progressed and Ron was struggling about letting me into such a personal aspect of his life. The dialogue was poignant and intimate and it made me realise how we were distancing ourselves from each other.

We saw the memory clinic nurse twice once in the autumn & once early this year 2018. She was much more thorough she spent time hearing our narrative. She initially agreed with the diagnosis of mild memory deficit.

In between the two visits other things began to show, Ron was beginning to ask me if I had just spoken, he admitted that he was hearing random voices. Then he started seeing things out of the corner of his eye, his balance was beginning to be affected. I did some research and it looked more like Lewy Bodies dementia, we returned to the memory clinic and she agreed and gave him this as a working diagnosis. We are still awaiting an appointment with the neurologist to confirm this but as the months go on I finally have to accept that he has dementia.

It is so hard on one hand Ron is still writing, he can still perform as a trainer, he is still great as a mentor, on the other hand a light is going dimmer in his eyes, his body is weaker, he has just had added a diagnosis of mild to moderate heart disease to his list. Some days he can complete cooking a meal, helping clean the house and then on other days he just retreats inside. He now has his own office where he spends increasing amount of his time. I think here he can be himself, there is no pressure, he can stare into space or watch loads of Netflicks, or write he doesn't have to perform or try to appear "normal" to us. I still find myself trying to catch him out, surely this isn't really happening. I increasingly find myself getting angry when he hasn't remembered anything I have asked him to do, I realise it's getting worse, dementia is slowly creeping in and taking over and there is nothing I can do about it.

Yet it's not all gloom we just managed a fantastic trip to Hong Kong where we were invited to train a very enthusiastic group about voices. Ron managed the flights, he did perform, where he stumbled I was quickly able to come in and keep the flow, yes there were differences, his energy levels were much lower, he didn't really want to engage much in social chit chat, he didn't want to be far from me. He did manage to get lost on one trip in the city when he wanted to return early than me to the hotel, but with a policeman's help found his way to the hotel. The best thing was we had time together on our own with no other interruption, time to be intimate and loving.

We can still have a life, that's a strong sentence, but there are times when I fear the future, already the house is becoming taken over with implements to help Ron, a bath chair, wheely trolleys, various aids for walking, my mind wants to resist are these really necessary. Selfishly I want them to go away yet they are allowing Ron his independence and confidence to do more, I see again the creeping in of dementia. The worst part is watching our youngest daughter face her emotions and see her Father changing. You can see her grieving already, this isn't all the time but when her guard is down. I suppose if I'm honest it is the same for me, I think I'm too coloured by my past work as a nurse working with older people with dementia to see a happy ending to all of this. I also struggle with the inner loneliness this condition creates not just in the person but for the whole family. Living in a remote area probably doesn't help that, but you can feel Ron drawing in, this isn't all the time but its noticeable and perhaps I do the same too we end up living side by side. One of the frustrations is even normal arguments are difficult, we had one the other day, he had forgotten most of it by the following day whilst I was still simmering with outrage.

The other frustration is with Lewy bodies he has a lot of restless legs and problems with sleep, sometimes this has a knock on effect on me not getting enough sleep, other times he gets up and disappears down stairs, only to return freezing cold several hours later and then there is the guilt that I had slept blissfully whilst he was standing vacant downstairs cold and lost. My answer is to "soldier on"' this is what I do, if nothing else my life has taught me to be self-reliant and just how capable I am, so I am looking after myself, I stubbornly stick to doing my running, yoga, meditation, swimming and at the moment reclaiming my garden at 28 Habost is consuming most of my time, getting my hands dirty, feeling physically tired fighting the nettles, thistles and docks, and don't even mention the horsetails is given me something really positive to focus on, fresh vegetables produced by me to feed us through the next year and hopefully an inner and outer strength which will help me in the future. It's also helping me prepare for moving back to Habost when we can build our extension so Ron has a house with no stairs. There is a future, I know he will fight all the way. I just need to find a way that allows us all to feel hopeful, because Ron has certainly not given up on hope and is fighting every step of the way.

Book One End Word

A multi-faceted brain attack,
Caused by an infusion of smoker's plaque?
Blocking our arteries like a beaver's dam,
Blowing up a storm within deepest calm

The short term thought,
Barred from long term memory,
Because lack of REM sleep,
Halts the neuron driven chemistry

That creates the space,
That is so elementary,
To make my thoughts,
Much more than temporary

Combative neurons so we're told
Tells us what our future holds,
But neurons can only have their way,
If they're allowed to fight and win the day

But to fight on when all say you cannot know,
The way the fights' results will go,
Makes us the winners no matter what,
Cause we did not surrender instead we fought

On to the end though death result,
For that is how the human spirit is built
For though we all must leave this human sphere,
We can walk in hope, or walk in fear